Yoga Builds Bones

Yoga Builds Bones

Easy Gentle Stretches
That Prevent Osteoporosis

Jan Maddern

ELEMENT

Boston, Massachusetts • Shaftesbury, Dorset
Melbourne, Victoria

First published in the USA in 2000 by
Element Books, Inc.
160 North Washington Street
Boston, Massachusetts 02114

Published in Great Britain in 2000 by
Element Books Limited
Shaftesbury, Dorset SP7 8BP

Published in Australia in 2000 by
Element Books Limited for
Penguin Books Australia Limited
487 Maroondah Highway, Ringwood, Victoria 3134

Library of Congress Cataloging-in-Publication data available
British Library Cataloguing in Publication data available

First Edition
10 9 8 7 6 5 4 3 2 1

Printed and bound in the United States

Cover design by Jane Ramsey
Book design by Faith Hague

ISBN 1-86204-821-5

Dedication

When my mother was first diagnosed with chronic osteoporosis in the late 90's, her world changed irrevocably. Yet despite the pain, disability and despair of this disease, she continued to be 100% responsible for managing her health. Today at age 77, she continues to read widely and explore all treatment options both orthodox and complementary. It has been her active participation in her treatment that has helped her to manage the disease. It was her determination to reclaim her independence that was the inspiration for this book. Thank you Maisie.

Special thanks. . .

To David of course—who shares my love of life and is always there for me.

To Ihab Nayal for capturing the strength and energy of yoga in his carefully drawn illustrations.

To my family and friends for their ongoing and loving support.

To Holly Schmidt at Element for her confidence in this book and to editor Jane Townswick for her sensitive editing.

To nutritionist Belinda Rennie for her valued input.

To the researchers at the National Osteoporosis Foundation, and the Yoga Research Center in the USA, and the Women's Health Resource Center, Australia.

To Margrit Segesman, Di Lucas and Lucille Wood at Gita International Yoga Australia for their refined wisdom which has stayed with me long after leaving the yoga school.

To the writers group in Dubai for their support when I lost the plot and was filled with self doubt, and for their test run of the yoga routines.

To all the yoga students in Dubai for their feedback and support.

To Telician for helping out with an additional last minute sketch.

Contents

Introduction

Strong bones are essential for maintaining good health at every stage of a woman's life. Primarily the result of weight-bearing exercise, good hormonal balance, sound nutrition, and genetic factors, normal healthy bone tissue is formed when old bone cells break down, become absorbed by the body, and are replaced by strong, healthy tissue that mineralizes and hardens. This process occurs at a fairly even rate, meaning that the amount of healthy bone anywhere in the body equals the amount that is broken down and absorbed.

When new bone cell production can't keep up with the breakdown of old bone cells, the result is a disease called osteoporosis. Characterized by thinning bones with low bone mass, increased fragility, and risk of fracture, osteoporosis has become a global problem in a world with rapidly aging populations. It is also a major health concern for women everywhere. By the time a woman is 35 years old, she has reached her "peak bone mass" and acquired as much bone density as she is ever likely to have. This is an indication of how well her bones will age throughout menopause.

The good news is that hatha yoga can help. Any woman who is willing to take responsibility for her total health and well-being, and regularly practice yoga weight-bearing postures with breathing exercises, is unlikely to have to suffer osteoporosis. Understanding the nature of this disease, the myths that surround it, and how hatha yoga can prevent it are the focus of this book.

Myths, Misconceptions, and Old Wives' Tales

Many widely held beliefs about osteoporosis simply aren't true. If you've ever had thoughts like these, you're not alone.

Myth #1: Osteoporosis is an inevitable part of aging.

Wrong. Bones do not have to grow old and crumble. With proper physical activity, you can apply enough force to your bones to maintain optimum calcium levels and good bone strength as long as you continue to be active.

Myth #2: Osteoporosis only affects old people.

Not so. Hormonal imbalances occur frequently in women as young as 35. Often linked to chemical pollutants in the environment, these imbalances can cause damage to the ovaries and lead to osteoporosis.

Myth #3: There are certain drugs you can take to prevent osteoporosis.

False. The drugs currently prescribed for osteoporosis produce only short-term benefits at best—no medication yet discovered can replace lost bone tissue, build new bone or prevent fractures over the long term.

Myth #4: Drinking milk and taking calcium supplements will protect against osteoporosis.

Wishful thinking. There is more calcium in products like canned fish, almonds, soy products, and green leafy vegetables than in dairy products, and the body absorbs these forms of calcium more easily. For example:

Food Item	Serving size	Calcium content mgs
Whole milk	8 oz	291
Canned sardines with bones	8 oz	992
Canned pink salmon	8 oz	480
Almonds	8 oz	640
Tofu (processed with calcium salts)	8 oz	600
Bok choy (raw)	8 oz	749

(Figures supplied by the Osteoporosis and Related Bone Diseases National Resource Center, Washington D.C.)

Note: Calcium supplements vary, but on an average they contain approximately 200 to 300 mgs per tablet. Reaching the daily recommended allowance means taking five or six tablets each day, which would be an expensive way of getting calcium. It is far cheaper and better nutritionally to obtain calcium from food sources like those listed above, which also contain other associated nutrients.

Myth #5: Taking estrogen can prevent bone loss.

Not the case. Osteoporosis can occur in young women with normal estrogen levels. While synthetic estrogen can sometimes slow down the rate of bone loss during the first stages of menopause, bone loss rates after that are the same for women who have never taken hormone replacement therapy.

Although synthetic estrogen appears to offer short-term benefits, it yields little long-term protection against bone fractures.

What causes osteoporosis?

Any and all of the following factors can contribute to the onset of thinning bones and an increased risk of fractures.

◆ *Insufficient hormone levels*

Estrogen, progesterone and parathyroid hormones are all necessary for efficient bone production. Progesterone stimulates bone formation, while synthetic estrogen temporarily retards the rate of bone loss during menopause. The parathyroid hormone maintains calcium levels in the blood and stimulates bone formation.

◆ *Lack of calcium*

If the vitamins and minerals needed for effective calcium absorption are not present, the body will excrete its reserves of calcium. (See chapter 1)

◆ *Little or no weight-bearing exercise*

Applying pressure to bones causes them to thicken and become stronger, and promotes the retention of calcium.

◆ *Certain medical conditions*

Surgical removal of the ovaries during a hysterectomy causes a rapid drop in estrogen levels and decreased bone density. Removing part of the digestive tract can result in less area of the body being available for calcium absorption. The eating disorder, anorexia nervosa, characterized by low calorie intake, poor nutrition and irregular menstrual cycles, can also increase the risk of thinning bones.

◆ *Genetic factors*

White and Asian women are more frequently affected by osteoporosis than black women, who tend to have thicker bones than women with lighter skins. Research has also indicated that women whose hair turns more than 50% gray before the age of 40 are four times as likely to develop osteoporosis as those whose hair does not turn gray by then.

Thin, short women do not have as much bone mass to begin with as larger women have, so they can't afford to lose much. Short, thin women also have less gravitational pull on their muscles, which means less work for their muscles and bones. Thus, these women are at risk of a decrease in bone mass over time.

Smokers usually eat less food than non-smokers, and often do not exercise regularly. Some studies show that women who smoke increase their risk of developing osteoporosis by 50%. Smoking is also harmful to the ovaries, and it can result in a drop in estrogen, causing earlier menopause. This means that a smoker loses bone over a longer period of time. Smoking also adversely affects the parathyroids, which control calcium balance in the body, causing calcium to be excreted from the bones over time. Therefore, a slender smoker is at greater risk of developing osteoporosis.

◆ *Differences in bone density*

Data from twin studies have shown that differences in bone density are partially due to genetic factors. Yet not all women who have thinning bones develop osteoporosis. Putting fluoride into water supplies was initially believed to contribute to strong bones, but while spinal density did increase during certain controlled fluoride studies, the rate of fractures also increased, due to diminished bone quality. In other words, high bone density does not necessarily protect against fractures, just as low bone density does not always result in fractures.

Additional Risk Factors

Although certain risk factors are not enough to predict a chance of suffering bone fractures by themselves, conditions like the following should not be ignored in regard to developing osteoporosis.

◆ *Poor postural stability and balance*
◆ *Low muscle strength*
◆ *Lack of body fat around the hips*
◆ *Cognitive disorders*
◆ *Excessive barbiturate or alcohol use that causes disorientation*
◆ *Impaired vision*

Early Detection

Often called a silent disease, osteoporosis can go unnoticed until a painful or debilitating fracture occurs. In the early stages, symptoms can include gum disease, loss of height, or developing a dowager's hump. Gum disease occurs when teeth bones become thin, and loose enough to irritate the gums, causing inflammation. Then the gums recede and form pockets, where bacteria can grow. A decrease in height can stem from compression of the vertebrae as bones become thinner, so it's a good idea to check your height every year after reaching the age of 40. Collapsed vertebrae can cause rounding of the top of the spine, a condition often called a dowager's hump. This can be accompanied by sharp pain, or be completely painless.

For accurate diagnosis, Bone Mineral Density (BMD) tests are used to measure the amount of bone mineral density, an important factor in determining bone strength. These tests are often recommended for people who go through early or surgical menopause, for fair-haired, thin women, and for people who have low levels of stomach acid. Both single and dual X-ray absorptiometry and quantitative computed topography can evaluate the risk for osteoporosis fractures with a 2% to 10% error rate. The potential for error is greatest in the lumbar spine, so testing the forearm and hip is preferable for both younger and older women. Many National Osteoporosis Organizations around the world recommend BMD testing if there is a history of previous fractures, low body weight, a family history of fractures, or cigarette smoking.

Hatha Yoga: Miracle Cure for Many Ailments

"Kathy," a chronic adult asthmatic for ten years, found walking up stairs impossible, even with the aid of a nebulator and daily doses of steroids. After attending a four-week retreat at a naturopathic yoga clinic, she was cured (and lost 22 pounds, and was able to throw away her prescription eyeglasses, as well). Today, she regularly practices the nutritional and yoga techniques she learned at the clinic, and has never experienced another asthma attack. What does hatha yoga involve, and how can it produce beneficial results like these?

Widely recognized as an effective, scientifically proven remedy for many of today's stress-based illnesses, hatha yoga de-stresses the body, mind and emotions, and promotes hormonal balance for maximum well-being and health. It includes breathing and meditation techniques that produce overall higher energy levels and a sense of emotional well being, improved muscular coordination and balance, mental concentration, relaxation, and inner peace of mind. It involves the whole person—physically, mentally, emotionally and spiritually, bringing the mind, body and emotions under control, so that the body can make use of its innate wisdom to heal itself. Smoking, obesity, anxiety and stress disorders and high blood pressure can all be improved by practicing hatha yoga. Even chronic ailments like asthma, arthritis, heart disease and degenerative disease can be improved or even cured by yoga.

For osteoporosis prevention, hatha yoga is one of the most superb forms of weight-bearing exercise known to mankind. Weight-bearing yoga postures increase strength and flexibility, stimulate bone development, and build bone strength evenly in both the upper and lower body. Yoga also contributes to healthy hormone levels and calcium balance, which limits bone loss, and works on the ovaries, which control estrogen/progesterone balance for bone remodeling. It affects the pituitary gland, which along with the ovaries and hypothalamus is thought to trigger the onset of menopause. With regular yoga practice, the endocrine glands function more effectively, which contributes to the formation and maintenance of strong, healthy bones. Yoga also works on the adrenals, keeping stress levels manageable and helping to avoid excessive calcium excretion. It works on the parathyroids, which maintain calcium levels in the blood. It improves the functioning of the pineal and adrenal glands, which at menopause produce an estrogen-like substance to counteract the body's falling levels of estrogen. Yoga improves strength, balance and coordination, helping to prevent falls, and it increases the supply of oxygen to all cells in the body for repair and regeneration.

The Endocrine Glands

Any discussion of hatha yoga would be incomplete without mentioning the endocrine glands, which are intricately linked to hormonal health and well-being. There are seven major endocrine glands in the body that affect health and well-being through the secretion of hormones. Hormones make us who we are, affecting moods, sleep patterns, energy levels, appetites, sexuality and even intelligence. Much of the activity and energy in the body centers around these glands because they control a multitude of functions.

1. The reproductive glands (ovaries in women, testes in men)
2. The adrenals (situated on top of the kidneys)
3. The Islets of Langerhans (in the pancreas)
4. The thymus (in the chest)
5. The thyroid and parathyroids (in the neck)
6. The pituitary (in the brain)
7. The pineal (also in the brain)

The Chakras

Corresponding to the seven endocrine glands are seven major sources of energy called chakras. We receive energy constantly from food, air, water and sunlight, all of which are necessary to keep us alive. Although the energy we take in from these sources is neutral, the energy we give out can be either negative or positive, depending on our thoughts and feelings. To understand this kind of energy transmission, think of a friend who always uplifts your spirits, compared to a person who drags you down with negative thoughts and feelings.

When the endocrine glands are over- or underactive, the resulting hormonal imbalance can cause all kinds of illnesses and inhibit the free flow of energy. Hatha yoga works to improve the functioning of the glands and to release energy blockages between the chakras, producing optimum health

The Endocrine Glands

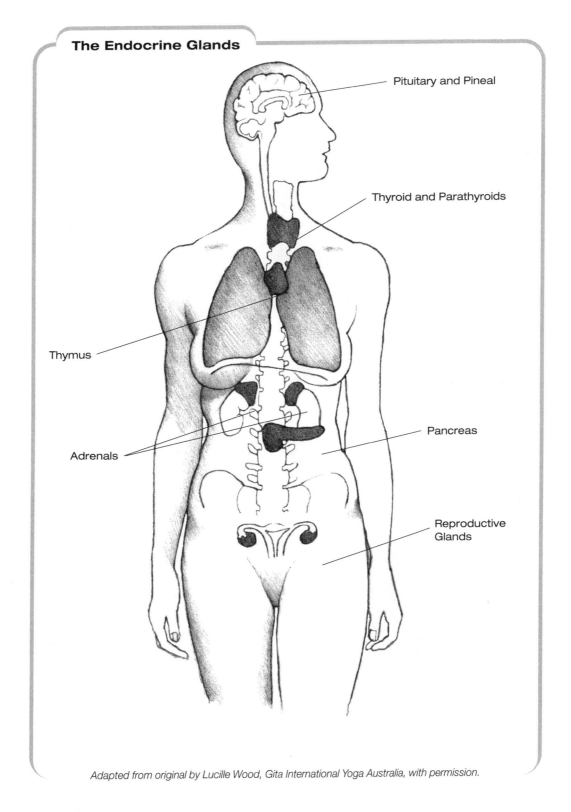

Pituitary and Pineal

Thyroid and Parathyroids

Thymus

Adrenals

Pancreas

Reproductive Glands

Adapted from original by Lucille Wood, Gita International Yoga Australia, with permission.

The Chakras

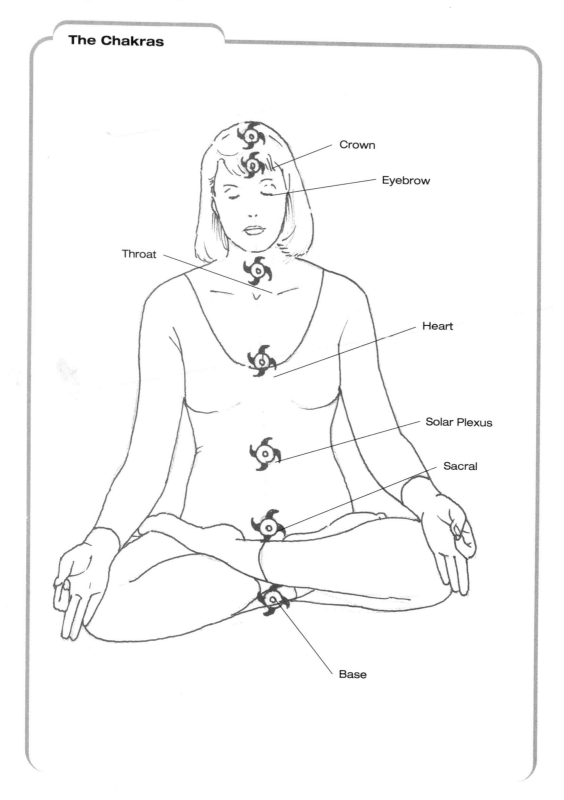

Crown

Eyebrow

Throat

Heart

Solar Plexus

Sacral

Base

and well-being. Each chakra relates to a certain endocrine gland and represents the positive personality characteristics shown below.

THE CHAKRA SYSTEM

Location	Color	Characteristics	Relates To:
1. Base of spine	Red	Primary force/vitality	Will to live—has a grounding effect
2. Sacral	Orange	Absorbs/distributes prana	Wise use of food, sex & money
3. Solar plexus	Yellow	Assimilation of food & energy	Emotional identification
4. Heart	Green	Discrimination in feelings	Empathy/ understanding of others
5. Throat	Sky Blue	Discrimination in thoughts	Mental creativity
6. Eyebrow center	Indigo	Center for intuition/ inspiration	Spiritual/personal ambition
7. Crown	Violet	Spiritual awareness	Reception of spiritual energies

How to Use This Book

Each routine in this book focuses on an endocrine gland or glands in a particular area of the body, and related yoga exercises that will help you build muscle strength, so it will be easier to do weight-bearing postures that build bone. You'll also learn postures that promote hormonal balance in the glands, for maintaining strong bones. You can practice in the comfort and privacy of your own home, and no special props or equipment are necessary. This book will help you:

◆ *Evaluate your own upper body strength*
◆ *Understand the role of calcium in building healthy bones*
◆ *Learn five different weight-bearing hatha yoga routines for retaining calcium and building muscle strength in your upper and lower body*
◆ *Improve the way your ovaries, adrenals and parathyroids function, to build and maintain stronger bones*
◆ *Improve the way your adrenal and pineal glands produce estrogen-like substances that offset falling levels of estrogen at menopause*
◆ *Alleviate five of the most common menopausal complaints: mood swings, lack of energy, inability to concentrate, weight gain and disruptive sleep patterns*

In short, the weight-bearing hatha yoga postures, breathing exercises, and meditation techniques in this book will enable you to take one hundred percent responsibility for your own health, so that your bones will remain strong and healthy throughout your life.

Note: The information in these pages is of a general nature. Osteoporosis is a serious degenerative disease, which in its worst forms can be life threatening. This book is not intended to replace the services of a trained health care professional, who can consult with you about matters relating to your own health or symptoms that require diagnosis and immediate attention.

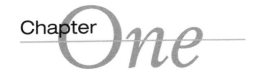

Chapter One

Beyond Calcium

Improving your knowledge of calcium and the factors that affect its absorption in the body will enable you to make lifestyle and dietary changes now to prevent thinning bones later in life. Adequate calcium absorption, hormonal balance and an effective weight-bearing routine are three of the most important factors in preventing osteoporosis. To test your current level of knowledge, take the following test, and check your answers at the end of this chapter before continuing.

Calcium Test *Answer True or False*

____ 1. Calcium's only role in the body is bone formation.

____ 2. Strong bones are the result of adequate calcium intake.

____ 3. The recommended daily allowance (RDA) of calcium for women over 40 years of age is 600 mg.

____ 4. No matter how much calcium you digest the ability to absorb calcium decreases with age.

____ 5. Calcium is absorbed with fats and oils.

____ 6. The Bantu tribe in Africa, with a lower than average intake of the RDA for calcium, have a higher rate of osteoporosis than Eskimos, who consume vast amounts of calcium.

____ 7. Regular exposure to the sun is necessary for the absorption of calcium.

____ 8. Fluoride, like calcium, is a bone-building mineral.

____ 9. Diets low in fat can cause thinning of the bones.

____ 10. Eating cheese of any kind will increase calcium levels.

_____ 11. All calcium supplements are equally well absorbed by the
       body.

_____ 12. Changes in the fingernails are an indicator of calcium
       deficiency.

Why Calcium Is So Important

Calcium is vital for proper brain function, blood clotting and muscle
contraction. A fluctuation as small as 3% in the body's calcium level can
result in severe debilitation, or even death. For this reason, the body is
equipped with an elaborate system of hormonal checks to make sure that
enough calcium is circulating in the bloodstream at all times. When blood
calcium levels fall, special hormones and glands respond immediately by
withdrawing whatever is needed from the storehouse in the bones. This
means that while calcium plays a major role in bone strength, it is also essential for maintaining other systems in the body.

Why Calcium Is Not a Cure-All

Women who take calcium can still lose bone, because a number of other
factors can prevent calcium from being absorbed and utilized by the body
effectively. Osteoporosis is not a disease that comes from a lack of dietary calcium, but rather, from excessive calcium loss caused by many factors.
Calcium is lost from bones faster than it is absorbed and utilized, no matter
how much is consumed in the diet.

It's important to understand that the type of calcium consumed affects
the body's ability to absorb and utilize it. For example, one of calcium's main
functions is to neutralize acid in the digestive system. If dairy products are
the body's main source of calcium, an acidic environment can occur in the
stomach. So while the body may be taking in plenty of calcium, the amount
in the bones and blood is constantly being used to neutralize this acid. Over
time, this can lead to a calcium deficiency and thinning bones.

Today, many health writers and nutritionists believe that calcium from
animal sources and dairy products is not the best source. Preferred sources
include soy products, vegetables and nuts, which are all easily absorbed and
do not create an acid environment in the stomach. If animal protein is a part
of the diet, nutritionists suggest eating no more than 35 grams per day or one
small serving of meat, fish, cheese or eggs. When you consider that having a
meal of eggs and bacon for breakfast supplies approximately 55 grams of protein, it's easy to understand that a typical Western diet is too high in animal
protein. An international nutrition journal recently published the results of
studies on protein consumption and its effect on calcium excretion. This
study concluded that a protein intake of 95 grams per day resulted in an

average calcium loss of 58mg. per day, representing a 2% loss of total skeletal calcium per year, or 20% per decade.

The negative effects of too much protein have been clearly demonstrated in patients who suffer from osteoporosis. Some medical scientists now believe that lifelong consumption of a high protein, acid-forming diet may be one of the primary causes of osteoporosis. On the other hand, while high protein consumption is a factor in the urinary excretion of calcium, it is also essential for healing fractures, which makes it necessary at times. Part of the reason for death or loss of independence experienced by the elderly after a hip fracture is protein-calorie malnutrition. Several studies have shown that protein supplementation following a hip fracture can decrease death rates and shorten convalescence.

The Importance of Calcium Absorption

Taking calcium supplements and eating calcium-rich foods is no good, unless they can be easily digested and absorbed by the body otherwise it may be excreted in the urine. Because excretion is a more important factor for determining calcium loss than poor absorption, it is critical to limit things like the following:

◆ *High protein, salt and acid-residue foods*

Dairy products can increase calcium excretion; unfortunately, many contemporary Western diets are high in protein and salt but low in calcium, which leads to increased calcium excretion and imbalance.

◆ *Coffee and cigarettes*

Drinking more than two cups of coffee per day and smoking cigarettes stimulates calcium excretion, reducing the amount of calcium in the blood. This stimulates the parathyroid gland to replace calcium lost from the blood by secreting a hormone that withdraws calcium from the bones.

◆ *Baking soda and aluminum cookware*

The combination of aluminum pots or pans and baking soda can lead to increased binding of phosphorous, excess excretion of calcium in the intestine, and inhibited absorption of fluoride in the intestine leading to bone loss.

◆ *Disease, illness and stress*

Any of these conditions will deplete the body's immediate supply of calcium, as well as its reserves, particularly if the stress is long-term, or chronic.

Factors Contributing to Poor Calcium Absorption

◆ *Lack of exercise (see why strength is so important, below)*

◆ *Lack of stomach acid*

◆ *A lack of certain nutrients*

For effective calcium absorption, the body needs phosphorus, magnesium, zinc, Vitamin C and D. There is evidence from recent studies to show that approximately 40% of the elderly who attend bone clinics are Vitamin D-deficient, as are 30% to 40% of patients with hip fractures. This scenario of the elderly spending increasing amounts of time indoors and becoming Vitamin D-deficient because of immobility is more and more common worldwide.

◆ *Foods high in phosphorous*

Eating foods with high phosphorous levels can cause calcium to form insoluble biochemical complexes, leading to inadequate absorption. Phosphorous-rich foods include cow's milk, fizzy drinks, processed or canned meats, such as ham, bacon, sausages or luncheon meats, processed cheeses, and packaged pastries and cakes. Always check food labels for phosphorous content before purchasing them.

◆ *Long-term use of antacids*

Antacids are now known to interfere with Vitamin D function and magnesium metabolism, both of which are necessary for calcium absorption. Antacids lower the acidity of fluids in the stomach, and habitual use may interfere with normal digestion and nutrient absorption.

◆ *Wheat and dairy products*

These foods can sometimes irritate the stomach and hinder digestion. If necessary, find out whether you are gluten- or lactose-intolerant. Many people are lactose-intolerant and have difficulty digesting milk.

◆ *Certain medications*

Some drugs inhibit calcium absorption because they lead to excretion of the vital nutrients required for calcium absorption. Antidepressants are known to accelerate the inactivation of vitamin D and increase Vitamin C excretion, as do certain barbiturates. Cholesterol-lowering drugs also decrease absorption of both calcium and Vitamin D, and they increase urinary excretion of calcium.

◆ *Certain medical conditions*

People who have chronic diarrhea absorb less calcium and lose more in their stools. The same is true for people who have had part of their digestive tracts removed. Check with your physician for medical factors like these that may affect your calcium absorption.

How to Improve Calcium Absorption

1. Check to see if you have adequate daily levels of the following minerals and nutrients necessary for calcium absorption: magnesium 300–350mg; zinc 15mg; phosphorous 23–50mg; Vitamin D 400–600IU; Vitamin C 60mg.

2. Increase your Vitamin C intake by eating two servings of fruit and five of vegetables per day, because Vitamin C helps the bones use available calcium in blood and soft tissues.

3. Calcium is absorbed together with fats and oils broken down by liver enzymes. If you have trouble digesting fatty foods and experience pain and indigestion after a fatty meal, you may want to read *The Liver Cleansing Diet*, by Dr. Sandra Cabot. In it, she explains the role of a healthy liver and offers a program for improving the ability of the liver to break down fats and improve calcium absorption.

4. Elderly people who lack adequate stomach acid can take betaine hydrochloride tablets before a protein-containing or calcium-containing meal to help increase calcium absorption. Alternatively, sipping a small glass of water containing a teaspoon of cider vinegar during every meal is also helpful. Check with your doctor first to establish if you have this type of deficiency.

5. Vitamin D helps bone remineralize, and it is stimulated by sunshine and regular outdoor exercise. It's a good idea to expose your face and arms to sunshine before applying any sun lotion between the hours of 8:00 AM and 4:00 PM. The amount of sunshine people need depends on the time of day, the season, where they live and how easily they experience sunburn. A good recommendation is to expose your face, hands and arms two or three times a week to 50 to 70% less sun than it would take to cause sunburn. For example, if you know you will get sunburn after 30 minutes of June sunlight at noon, try to expose your skin to a maximum of only 5 to 10 minutes of sun, without sunscreen.

6. Consider taking a blood test for Vitamin D if you are over the age of 50. Have this test done in mid-winter, because there can be a 3% bone loss in winter, related to Vitamin D deficiency. If your body can make enough vitamin D during summer, it can be stored in fat tissues for use during winter. Alternatively, consider taking a Vitamin D supplement. While the increase in bone density from trials with Vitamin D are small (around 1% to 2% over two years), this may be enough to take you out of the risk range for fractures.

7. Since foods containing oxalic acid (found in artichokes, spinach, rhubarb and chocolate) impede calcium absorption, eat these only in moderation. If you think you're a "chocoholic," buy the most expensive and best quality chocolate you can afford, and eat it as an occasional treat.

Why Strength Is So Important

Most osteoporosis fractures occur in the upper body, where many women are physically weakest. In order to build bone and maintain calcium levels in this area, the arms and the upper spine must have enough strength to push against gravity and support the body's weight. Astronauts, who are unable to do weight-bearing exercises against gravity, lose bone mass rapidly in space. Hence, current space research is increasingly involved in understanding the prevention of osteoporosis. This research indicates that the force exerted on the body when it meets the ground is what keeps muscles and bones strong in the lower body. When this happens, mechanical and bio-electrical signals are transmitted to the bone, causing it to retain calcium and thicken in response to use. The key is to determine how individuals can "load" their bodies to maintain muscle and bone strength. Since our muscles generate their own forces, we are limited by how strong our muscles are. The bottom line is that if you do not have enough muscle strength, you cannot exert a high enough force on your bones to increase bone mass. As we age, our levels and intensity of physical activity can decrease, muscle strength can decline, and therefore our ability to load our bones can decrease. The result can be weaker bones with less density, which are more prone to fractures. This need not be the case, however, if we are prepared to exercise so we can maintain muscle and bone strength throughout our lives.

Self-Assessment for Upper Body Strength

To test your upper body strength, try these three simple exercises below. If you are 40 years plus, don't be surprised if your arms wobble when you attempt the test for upper body strength. You may be unable to complete and maintain the positions for the time period stated. Even women who walk regularly, do aerobic exercise or play tennis or squash find these exercises difficult. This is because they are used to bearing weight mainly on their legs, and they have less strength in their upper bodies. Use this assessment for upper body strength as a diagnostic tool, to become aware of where your upper body needs to be strengthened. Take note when your body is straining, which indicates a weakness in the muscles and joints. If there is too much strain or discomfort, discontinue the exercise and go to the next one.

Exercise 1: Inverted Push Up

1. Stand with your legs wide apart, lean forward, and place your out-stretched hands on the floor, a shoulder width apart. Turn your hands inward and spread your fingers wide.

2. Push your hips up to the ceiling, and have the body in a strong inverted "V" position.

3. Move your weight forward onto your hands, bend your elbows, and touch your nose to the floor, if you can.

Inverted Push Up

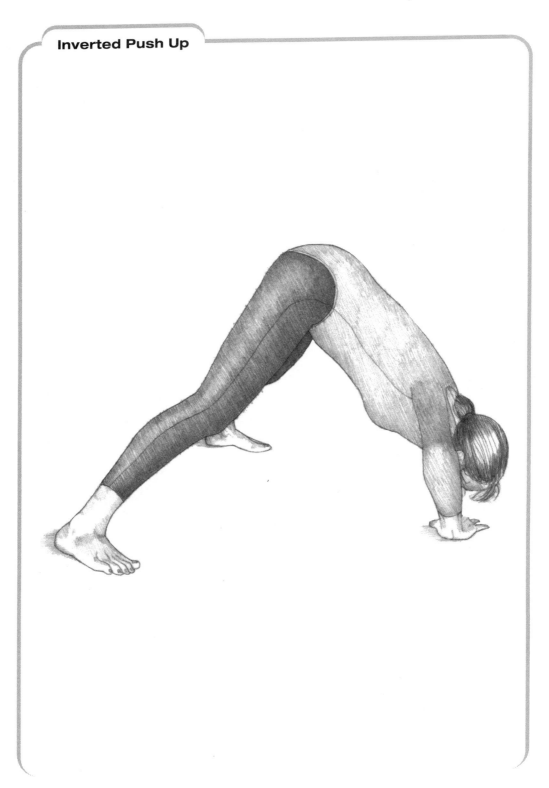

4. Keep your hips high, toward the ceiling in the "V" position, and breathe deeply in and out through your nose for two breaths.

5. To return, straighten your elbows, and push your weight back into your heels with your arms and legs straight.

6. Stretch and lengthen your spine, by pushing your head further through the shoulders and the hips up to the ceiling.

7. Repeat seven times, if possible, then relax onto your stomach, with your hands loosely by the side of your body, and breathe deeply and slowly for a few minutes.

Exercise 2: Seated Fish

1. Sit on the floor, with your legs stretched out in front of you, and your palms flat on the floor beside your thighs.

2. Adjust your fingers, so that they point away from your body.

3. Take your weight on your hands, and lift your hips as high as possible toward the ceiling, and balance on your arms and hands with your elbows locked.

4. Pinch your shoulder blades together, drop your head back, and point your toes to the floor for support.

5. Breathe slowly in and out through your nose, and hold this position for three breaths.

6. To return, lower your hips to the seated position, and take a deep slow breath.

7. Repeat this position two more times, and visualize your wrists, forearms and upper arms becoming stronger.

8. Next, hold this position steady; raise one leg in the air, and balance, while taking three slow breaths. Return to the seated position.

9. Repeat the raised-leg position twice with each leg.

10. Return your hips to the floor, and lie down, letting your breath come easily in and out through your nose. Have your feet apart and your palms facing upward, in an open position. Lie quietly, while watching your chest rise and fall, and deepen the breath.

Seated Fish

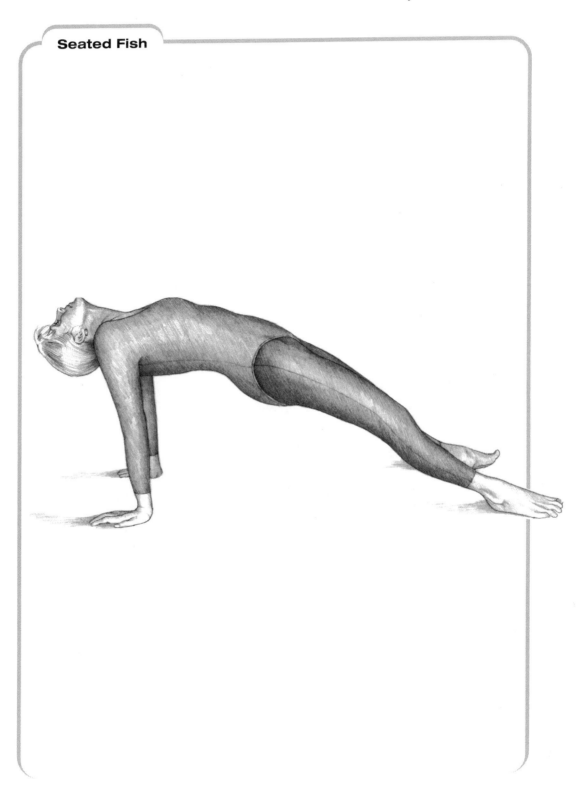

Exercise 3: Balanced Hip Lift

1. Sit on the floor, with your legs extended.

2. Roll onto your left hip, and place both palms flat on the floor in front of your hips.

3. Cross your right ankle over your left, so that the toes of your right foot gently rest on the floor.

4. Take your weight onto your hands, and lift your hips as high as possible to the ceiling.

5. Push the toes of your right foot firmly into the floor to hold your balance.

6. Inhale, and extend your right arm up to the ceiling. Look up at your extended hand.

7. Pull your right shoulder and hip back, and focus on the strength of your left arm supporting your body weight.

8. Breathe slowly in and out of your nose for three breaths, and return your hips to the floor.

9. Repeat this lift and stretch two more times on your left side, and then roll onto your right hip and repeat it three times on the other side.

10. To release, lie on your back with your feet flopped apart, and your palms upward. Rest for a few moments, and breathe deeply and slowly.

If you realize, after completing these exercises, that your upper body is weak in muscle strength and possibly bone strength, now is the time to correct the situation. Perhaps there is weakness in your wrist and ankle joints, which are unable to support your body's weight for very long without discomfort. Upper body, weight-bearing exercises work to strengthen the wrist and ankle joints, and at the same time, they help prevent stiffness and soreness to these joints as we age. More importantly, medical science has been unable to successfully replace either of these joints in the body, because they are so complex and capable of such a wide range of movement. If these joints stiffen or are damaged as we age, our range of activities will be severely limited. Therefore, it's imperative to strengthen them by putting weight on these joints, and by rotating them through a full range of movement, for increased flexibility. With regular weekly practice, this type of weight-bearing exercise will effectively build muscle and bone strength in the upper body over time. As muscle strength builds, your arms will be able to support these positions for a longer period of time.

Balanced Hip Lift

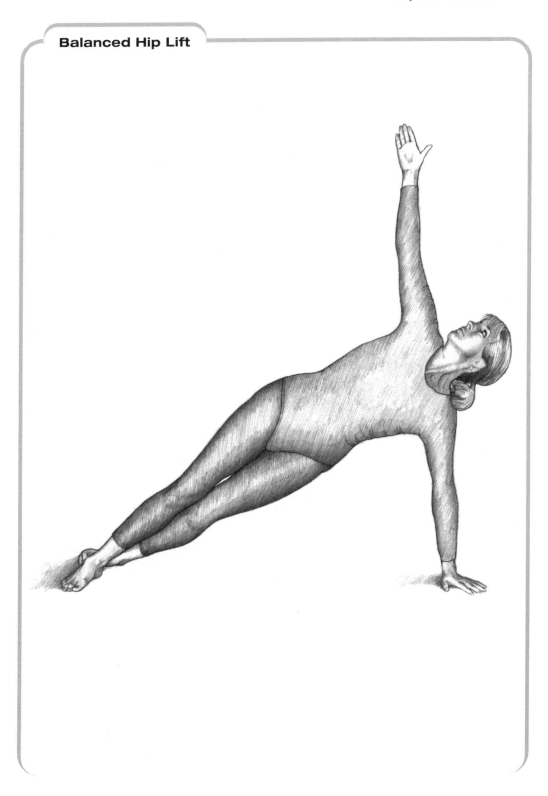

The Correlation between Yoga and Osteoporosis

Every day, yoga teachers around the world see many people who do not show the predicted 1 in 4 incidence of osteoporosis commonly found in post-menopausal women. They report seeing little or no incidence of osteoporosis in their regular students. Those who have detected early signs of osteoporosis, and improved their calcium intake and practice of specific bone-building postures, have reported increased bone densities. These are, in some cases, closer to those in a 35-year-old woman, rather than someone who has reached the age of 55.

Take the case of "Amy," who at the age of 50 had been teaching and practicing yoga for many years. One day, after feeling a twinge in her back, she went to her doctor. A bone mineral density test revealed the beginnings of bone thinning in her lower spine, and hormone replacement therapy was prescribed. Amy's periods started again, she experienced severe bouts of hemorraging, and her blood pressure increased dramatically. By the age of 52, she had to have a hysterectomy. She stopped taking HRT, because while it had initially improved her bone density, it had also created more life-threatening problems. Amy had studied Chinese medicine, and resorted to her textbooks for a holistic approach to building bone density. She increased the number of weight-bearing yoga postures she did each day, walked, and did water aerobics on a regular basis. To improve her digestion and absorption of calcium, she decreased her consumption of all the acid-producing foods, including red meat, dairy products, coffee and alcohol. In addition, she increased her consumption of alkaline-producing foods, such as fruits and vegetables. Because Chinese medicine views the kidneys as responsible for bone health, she increased her consumption of foods that helped kidney function, including seaweed products, black beans, and sardines. She now regularly takes a multivitamin supplement, and works to improve her digestion system with plenty of alkaline-producing foods. Today, at age 67, Amy has the bone density of a person much younger and has never had an osteoporosis fracture.

While most of the scientific community only sits up and takes notice of random, double-blind, placebo-type studies, this kind of observational evidence from yoga teachers around the world cannot be discounted. Numerically, the number of yoga students worldwide is small, but statistically, the high percentages of older yoga students who do not suffer osteoporosis are highly significant. There is startling evidence from yoga teachers throughout the world supporting the hypothesis that the regular practice of hatha yoga prevents osteoporosis. Therefore, this observational evidence must stand, until the scientific community recognizes the high correlation between the two and begins to conduct controlled studies.

Standing Spine Twist

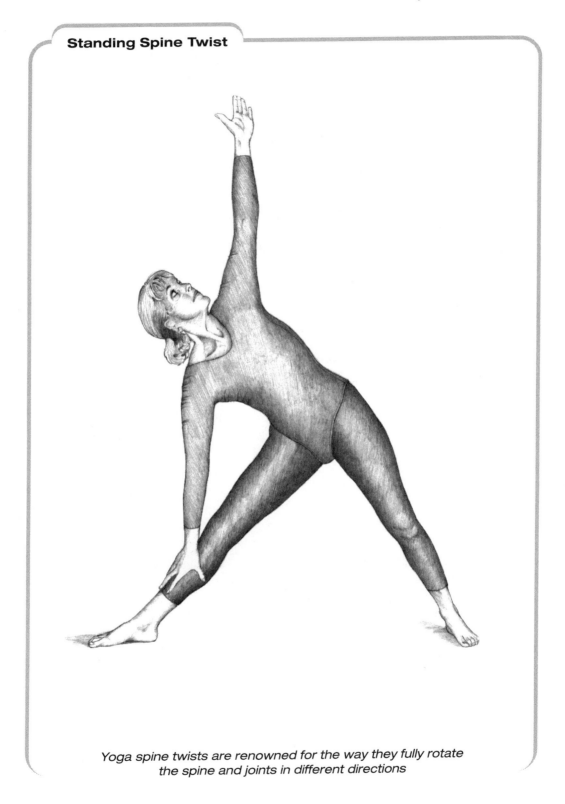

*Yoga spine twists are renowned for the way they fully rotate
the spine and joints in different directions*

Why Such a Strong Correlation?

Hatha yoga is so successful in preventing osteoporosis because of the following factors, each of which is discussed more fully, below.

- *Fully rotates the joints and spine*
- *Strengthens muscles*
- *Builds bone strength through weight-bearing postures*
- *Balances the glands responsible for estrogen, progesterone, calcium, and adrenaline levels, all of which contribute to bone strength*
- *Increases oxygen for the repair and regeneration of bone cells*
- *Improves focus, concentration, coordination and balance to prevent falls*

Yoga Rotates the Joints and Spine

In many yoga postures, the spine and joints are rotated fully in different directions. These movements, which increase the circulation to the joint and decrease stiffness and pain, are similar to methods used by physiotherapists working on a damaged joint. They are equally beneficial to a healthy joint.

Yoga Strengthens Muscles

Warm-up yoga stretches focus on building muscle strength in specific parts of the body, and on improving flexibility in all of the joints. Strong, deep stretching exercises throughout the whole body enable students to develop enough strength to exert the force necessary for building strong bones. Yoga builds strength in the upper arms, shoulders and back muscles, so that students can support their own weight in inverted postures. It also builds strength in the upper thigh muscles, so that students can support their weight on one leg at a time.

Yoga Is Weight-Bearing

Other forms of weight-bearing exercise, such as walking, dancing, jogging and aerobics, bear weight mainly through the legs. Yoga is one of the few exercise systems in which weight is borne not only in the legs, but in the upper body and arms, as well. Inverted weight-bearing yoga postures, like the Crane on page 26, take the whole body weight on the bones of the arms, wrists, shoulders and hands to strengthen them. At the same time, they relieve tension in the shoulders and neck and improve balance and co-ordination, which are important for preventing falls and fractures in elderly people. Yoga develops spinal strength and maintains the health and integrity of the spine, which then allows the body to bend backward and forward in weight-bearing postures. Over time, these postures can help prevent curvature of the spine and compression of the vertebrae.

Pelvic Floor Lift

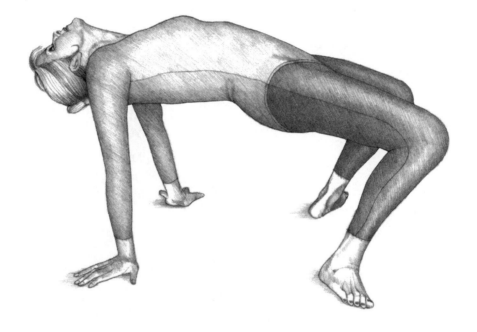

*This type of pelvic lift posture builds muscle and bone strength
equally in both the upper and lower body*

The Crane

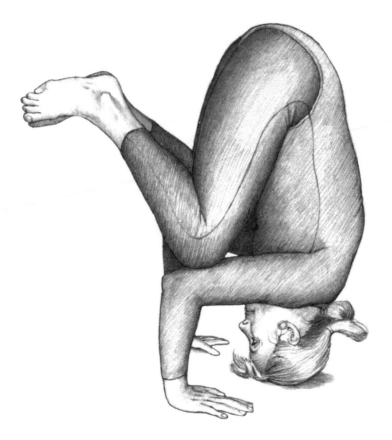

*Inverting the body weight onto the hands and head
stimulates bone strength in the arms, shoulders and spine.*

Yoga Balances Glands

What is least understood about yoga is its amazing effect on the glandular system, which controls our moods, appetites, sleep patterns, sexuality and intelligence. Prior to and throughout menopause, the regular practice of hatha yoga promotes a smooth transition by enhancing hormonal balance. It balances the glands that trigger menopause (ovaries, hypothalamus and pituitary) and those that take over the production of estrogen-like substances at menopause. It balances the glands responsible for our calcium levels and bone strength. When all of the glands are working properly, premature aging—including bone loss—is prevented.

Yoga Improves Oxygen Supply

Deep, rhythmic breathing or "pranayama" is an integral part of the practice of yoga. Students are taught to breathe deeply throughout the postures and to apply many different breathing techniques to calm the emotions and still the mind in preparation for meditation. This deep breathing increases oxygen to nourish, repair and regenerate the cells of the body, so important in bone remodeling.

Yoga Improves Focus and Concentration

The combination of deep, rhythmic breathing and the balancing yoga postures (asanas) also has a very powerful effect on restoring concentration and focus. For elderly people, who often complain of poor memory, concentration, and balance (often leading to falls), yoga offers one of the safest, most effective ways to prevent these falls. For yoga students of all ages, the increased focus developed during class can be applied outside class to the life goals that are important to each of us.

Should You Join a Yoga Class?

While this book gives you guidance on a number of simple stretches and postures, you can benefit greatly by joining a weekly yoga class, where you can learn to:

◆ *Perfect the postures*
◆ *Increase variety and avoid boredom*
◆ *Advance to stronger postures with qualified instruction*
◆ *Enjoy the energy and inspiration within a group of like-minded people*
◆ *Receive professional help, if problems occur*
◆ *Appreciate the holistic approach of physical, mental, emotional and spiritual aspects of yoga*

Answers to the Calcium Test

1. *False.* While 99% of the calcium in the body is located in the bones and only 1% in the blood, calcium is vital to brain function, transmission of nerve impulses, blood clotting, enzyme regulation and muscle contraction.

2. *False.* Strong bones are the result of many factors, and adequate calcium is but one of them. Others include genetic factors, hormonal balance, the level of weight-bearing exercise, the body's ability to absorb calcium, the presence or absence of lifestyle factors that hinder absorption and the availability of other bone building nutrients, such as Vitamin D, magnesium, phosphorus and zinc.

3. *False.* It varies between organizations and writers, and is related to both age and lifestyle. On average, the RDA for pre-menopausal women is 1000 to 1200mg, but 1500mg for menopausal and postmenopausal women. Some doctors recommend 4000 mg for periods of prolonged stress. We must remember that the RDA are estimates only, based on the best scientific data of levels of essential nutrients that would meet the needs of 95% of a healthy population. The RDA does not indicate the required level of nutrient intake or the minimum levels of nutrient needed.

4. *True.* Calcium is absorbed effectively when there is sufficient hydrochloric acid in the stomach. The body's ability to produce sufficient hydrochloric acid decreases with old age, and this will hinder calcium absorption. An inability to produce sufficient acid in the stomach is a condition called hypo-chlorhydria and this can be diagnosed and treated by your health practitioner.

5. *True.* Bile salts are created by the liver and stored in the gallbladder. When fatty foods enter the upper portion of the small intestine called the duodenum, a hormone is released that stimulates the gallbladder to release bile to the duodenum. Bile salts and water create a solution that emulsifies fats and oils, and calcium is absorbed together with the fats and oils.

6. *False.* Protein-rich foods, such as meat and fish, form the basis of the Eskimo diet. These foods in excess are acid forming, and the body cannot tolerate substantial changes in acid levels in the blood. It neutralizes the acid with calcium, which is withdrawn from the bones. Also, an excessive intake of animal protein, with its high phosphate content, increases urinary excretion of calcium and may promote or accelerate bone loss. The difference between the Bantu tribes and Eskimos is that the Eskimo diet is high in animal protein and the Bantu tribe is low in animal protein and high in vegetable protein, which is less acid-forming. Therefore, the Eskimos have the higher incidence of osteoporosis.

7. *True.* While the risk of skin cancer from too much exposure to the sun is real, a moderate amount of sunshine is needed to produce Vitamin D, which is essential for increased calcium absorption.

8. *False.* The addition of fluoride to water supplies may increase bone mass, but it fails to increase bone strength and the fracture rate incidence is actually

increased in non-vertebral bone by fluoride, particularly hip fractures. The use of fluoride is also associated with undesirable side effects, including gastro-intestinal inflammation and weakening of bone formation.

9. *True.* The amount and type of fat you consume affects calcium absorption; the preferred forms of fat are those found in fish and olive oils. If fat consumption is too low, calcium absorption is depressed because calcium is absorbed with fats and oils. This has been a major criticism of fat-free diets among women, particular in young women, when it leads to extreme thinness and eating disorders. Among young women, anorexia nervosa is associated with low bone mass, bone loss and osteoporosis, because anorexic teenagers often cease ovulating. This results in decreased levels of both estrogen and progesterone, and over time, leaves anorexics more at risk at menopause, when they have less bone density to draw on during the first few years of rapid bone loss. Sadly, the correction of this disease does not appear to fully return bone mass to normal levels. In older women, the amount of body fat also affects bone loss. Fat cells take over the production of estrogen-like substances at menopause, when bone loss is greatest. Too little body fat in older women can reduce this production of estrogen-like substances to offset the naturally falling levels of estrogen from the ovaries at menopause.

10. *False.* Certain cheeses, like low-fat ricotta, are very high in calcium, as is Parmesan, but the denser, heavier cheeses, such as Parmesan, are also higher in fat content. Also, many processed cheeses, such as cheddar, are high in phosphorous, whereas an unprocessed cheese, like ricotta, is not. While a certain amount of phosphorous is needed for calcium absorption, along with magnesium, heavy consumption of phosphorous-rich foods cause calcium to form insoluble biochemical complexes, leading to inadequate absorption of whatever calcium is consumed. Check the labels of packaged goods and avoid sodium phosphate, potassium phosphate, phosphoric acid, pyrophosphate and polyphosphate.

11. *False.* Calcium is reasonably well absorbed in any form, but some forms are better than others. For example, the best forms of calcium supplements are calcium amino acid chelate or citrate, which are approximately twice as well absorbed as calcium carbonate. Processed oyster shells and animal bones are often used to make calcium supplements, but much of this calcium is in the form of calcium phosphate. This is one of the least easily absorbed forms of calcium. Also, some calcium supplements include other minerals needed to enhance absorption, so check that in meeting your RDA for calcium that you are not over-dosing on the other nutrients in the supplement. You will need to consult a doctor about the use of calcium supplements if you have kidney stones, are taking diuretics, or have been diagnosed as hypertensive.

12. *False.* Contrary to popular belief, fingernail changes are not necessarily indicators of calcium deficiency. Breaking, brittle, or spotty nails may also be due to a lack of iron, zinc or essential fatty acids.

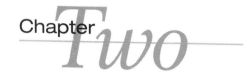

Chapter *Two*

Getting Started

The following stretches are designed to warm the body before attempting any of the routines that follow. They will stretch your spine, shoulders, hips and hamstring muscles effectively. In all stretches, breathe in and out evenly through your nose, unless otherwise stated. Never attempt any of the routines in the five following chapters without first spending a few minutes warming up your body with some of these easy stretches.

Complete the warm-up with seven rounds of full yoga breath, as shown on pages 43–47.

1. TABLETOP

Benefits: This stretch releases stiffness and soreness in the spine, shoulders and hamstrings, while strengthening the stomach muscles that support the spine.

Focus: on pushing up from the pads of your hands on the outward stretch, and pushing your hips high in the air to lengthen throughout the whole spine. Also, focus on tightening your stomach muscles in the rounded stretch, as you push your hands further through your feet.

1. Stand with your legs wide, feet turned out slightly to the side, and your arms extended at shoulder height.

2. Bend forward until your back is parallel to the floor, and hold this position for three breaths, while tightening your stomach muscles. Keep your legs locked and strong.

3. Stretch your arms forward and hold them parallel to the floor while breathing slowly three times.

Tabletop

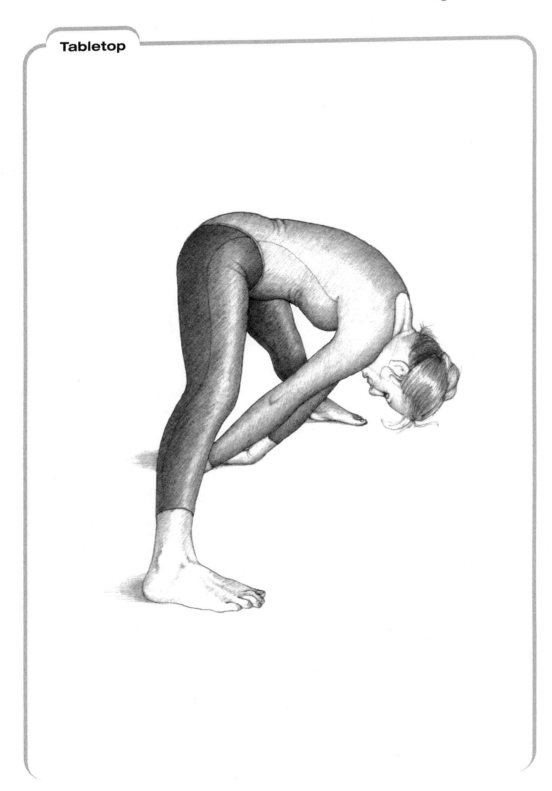

4. Place them on the floor, so that your body is now in an inverted "V" shape.

5. Push your head through your shoulders, and stretch through your spine, by pointing your hips to the ceiling. Keep your legs straight, to stretch the hamstrings.

6. Take three slow breaths in and out through your nose.

7. Place the back of your palms on the floor, and push them as far through your legs as you can, so your spine is rounded. Breathe three times, slowly.

8. Repeat this movement of stretching and rounding of the spine three times, and hold each stretch for three breaths.

2. ROTATED TABLETOP

Benefits: This stretch rotates the spine, hips and neck to a point of resistance to increase circulation to the joints and release stiffness.

Focus: on lengthening through the front of your body on inhalation, and softening and squeezing into the groin on exhalation.

1. Stand with your feet wide apart, bend forward, and place your outstretched hands on the floor, palms down, as in the previous exercise.

2. Walk your hands in a wide circle over to your right foot, and place them on the outside of your right foot, if you can. If this is not possible, place them on the outside of your calf muscles. Keep your knees straight, if possible.

3. Inhale slowly, lengthening through your spine, then exhale, and lower your head along your right leg squeezing into the groin.

4. Repeat for three breaths, lengthening in the spine each time on inhalation, and feel the stretch in your hamstrings on exhalation.

5. Return, by walking your hands in a wide circle back to the center.

6. Walk your hands over to the outside of your left leg, and repeat, while holding the position for three breaths.

Rotated Tabletop

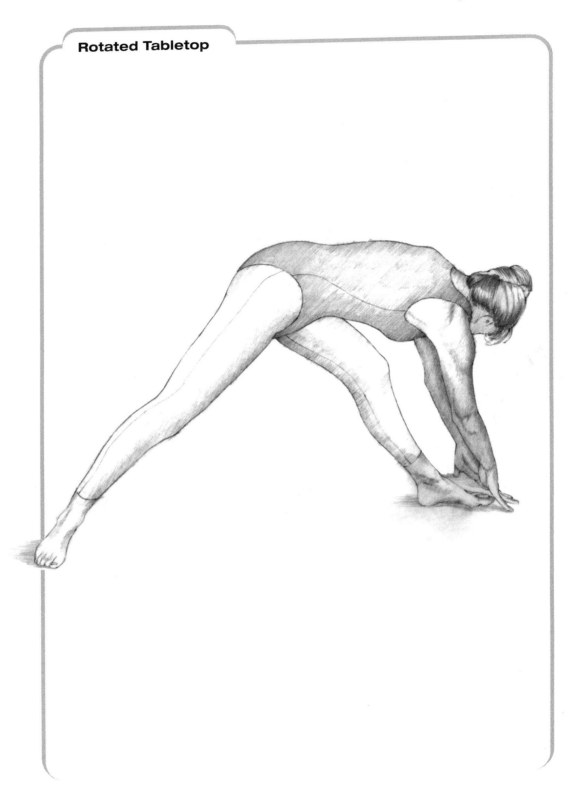

3. SQUATS

Benefits: When the head is lower than the heart in this stretch, circulation to the brain is improved, for clearer thinking. The body does not have to push against gravity to move the blood to the brain. The weight of the head lengthens the muscles around the vertebrae, so that the spine can release trapped muscles and nerves, and both circulation and energy to this area improve.

Focus: on feeling the stretch from your hamstrings, right through to the whole of your spine, as you straighten your legs.

1. Stand with your legs hip-width apart, lean forward and place your clenched fists on the floor inside your feet. Squat down, keeping your fists inside your feet, and your elbows inside your knees.

2. Straighten your legs, pushing the hips high to the ceiling, but keep your fists firmly on the floor. Drop your head down. Feel the stretch in your hamstrings.

3. Repeat this squat and straightening of the thighs seven times.

Squats

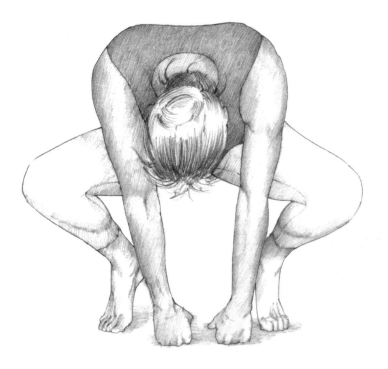

4. SHOULDER SWINGS

Benefits: This stretch opens up the shoulder joint and rotates the hip, shoulder and neck to a point of resistance, to increase the circulation to these joints and release stiffness.

Focus: on rotating your hip and shoulder joint as far as you can to each side. Feel the rotation and stretch of your whole spine.

1. Stand with your legs wide apart and inhale taking the arms in a wide circle above your head. Release your arms on exhalation, and place both palms firmly on the floor, a shoulder-width apart.

2. Inhale and, looking to the right, swing your right arm in a wide circle to the right as far as possible, pulling your right shoulder and right hip back.

3. Exhale, and return your right palm to the center.

4. Inhale and, looking to the left, swing your left arm in a wide circle to the left as far as possible, pulling your left shoulder and hip back. Exhale and return.

5. Repeat this swinging movement seven times to each side, inhaling on the stretch and exhaling on the return to the center, using steady, even breaths.

Shoulder Swings

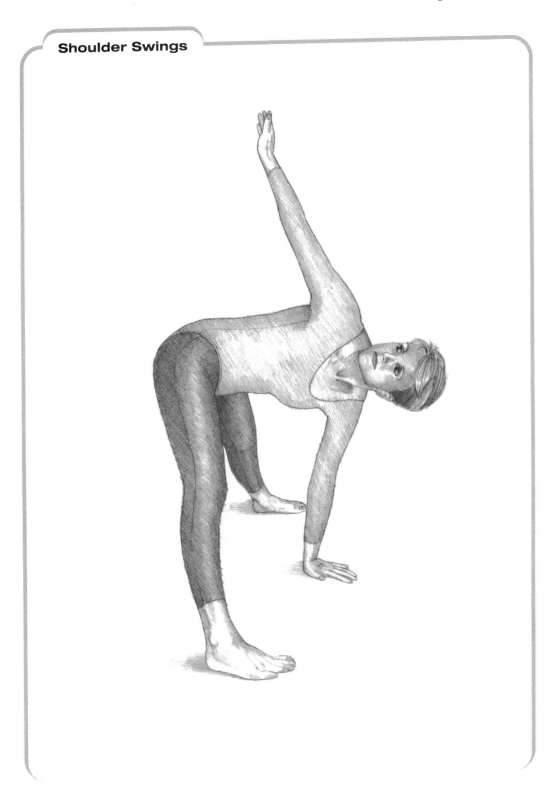

5. SEATED SPINE STRETCH

Benefits: This stretch supports the body weight on the wrists, and strengthens the wrist joint and bones. It releases tension throughout the spine and shoulders. Dropping the head back creates a lock on the parathyroids in the neck, which regulate calcium balance. Stretching through the front of the body physically opens up the emotional center in the solar plexus, so that the emotional energy can flow freely without blockages. This is an excellent stretch to start the day free of tension, both physically and emotionally.

Focus: on lengthening through the front of your thighs and keeping the buttocks off your heels by arching your back strongly. On an emotional level, focus on an openness through your stretched solar plexus, and breathing out any negative emotions of the week with the outward breath, including any feelings of irritation, frustration, resentment, fear or anxiety.

1. Kneel on the floor, with the front of your feet flat on the floor. Take hold of both calf muscles and pull them outward.

2. Sit between your heels inside your calf muscles, with the buttocks touching the floor between your hips.

3. Lean back and place your palms flat on the floor, about 6" away from your heels. Point your fingers toward your heels.

4. Inhale and lift your hips, and arch your back as high as possible.

5. Drop your head back and pinch your shoulder blades together, and focus on lifting your hips and stretching the front of your thighs.

6. Breathe slowly for seven breaths.

7. To return, lower your hips and sit between your heels again.

8. Repeat twice more, holding the position for seven breaths.

Note: As your thigh muscles become stronger, you may wish to make this a more challenging stretch. If so, then tuck your toes under, and then lift your hips, while holding for seven breaths, and feel the stronger stretch along your thighs.

Seated Spine Stretch

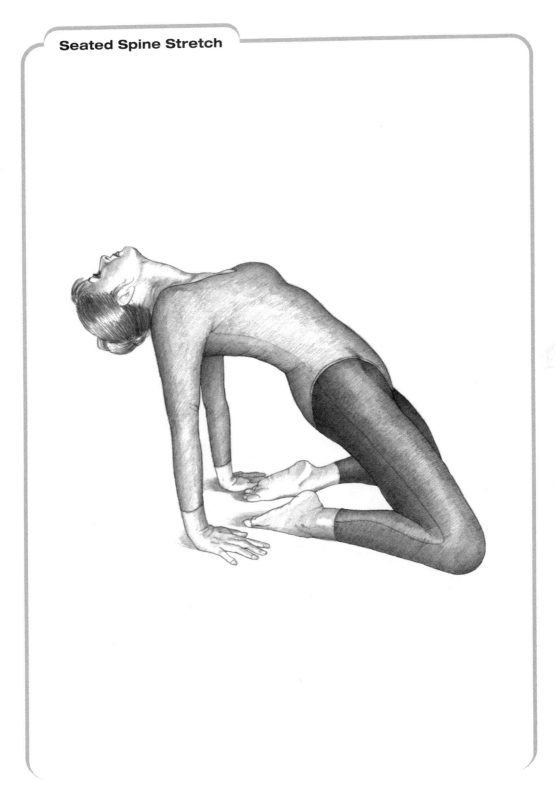

6. SPINE CURL

Benefits: Releases stiffness and soreness in the shoulders, lower back and in the neck.

Focus: on stretching your chin forward as far as possible to lengthen through your neck and spine.

1. Lie on the floor and bend your right knee into your chest, and clasp it with both hands.

2. Inhale, then exhale, and bring your chin onto your right knee, and hold.

3. Exhale, and lower your head to the floor. Repeat three times, change sides, and repeat three times on the other side.

4. Next, clasp both knees to your chest.

5. Inhale, then exhale, and bring your chin between your knees, and hold. Exhale, and return your head to the floor. Repeat three times.

Spine Curl

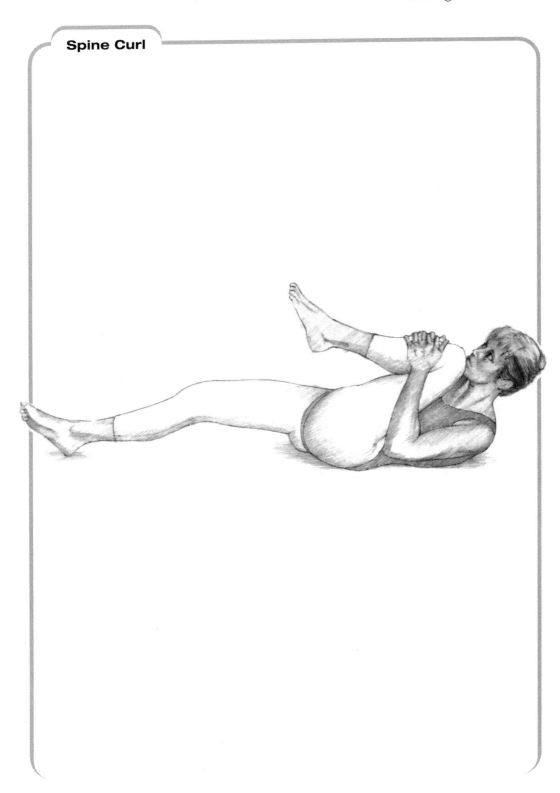

7. FULL YOGA BREATH

The full yoga breath (FYB) is used throughout many of the postures because it uses all of the lung capacity for maximum energy. Babies automatically practice full yoga breathing because this is the way we were born to breathe. The next time you see a baby, watch how it breathes, to see a FYB in perfect action. Unfortunately, as adults, we have forgotten how to breathe naturally and effortlessly, because of poor posture and rushing to meet deadlines. Most of us take breathing for granted and do not consciously breathe using the entire lung capacity.

Very few people are aware of the multitude of benefits of deep rhythmic breathing and of how crucial it is to our health and well-being. Deep breathing nourishes every cell in the body for repair and regeneration, and prevents premature aging. Germs cannot live in pure oxygen, so the immune system is strengthened and fewer infections occur. Improved oxygen levels in the blood increase metabolic rate and energy levels. The full use of all muscles of the abdomen and upper chest in deep rhythmic breathing releases tension in the neck and shoulder area, and releases stress naturally. The increased oxygen to the brain promotes clear and focused thinking, which improves balance and concentration, to prevent falls and fractures in later life.

What does oxygen deprivation do to the body?

Many people are deprived of oxygen on a daily basis through shallow or erratic breathing. They breathe from the upper chest instead of down in the abdomen, where the large diaphragm muscle sits. It is the movement of the diaphragm muscles that allows the whole chest to expand and fill with air. When only the upper chest muscles are used to breathe, the neck and shoulder muscles become strained throughout the day. The breath can sometimes feel as if it is stuck and sighing increases, as stiffness sets in around the upper chest. Long-term ill-health can occur because of incorrect breathing patterns, which can:

◆ *Deplete the body of energy*
◆ *Lower resistance to disease*
◆ *Increase stress levels because of a build-up of carbon dioxide, which irritates the cells and increases nervous tension*
◆ *Thicken the blood and slow circulation, making it sluggish*

How do incorrect breathing patterns show up?

◆ *Inability to concentrate*
◆ *Lack of energy*
◆ *Chronic tiredness*
◆ *Lack of motivation*
◆ *Irritability*

Full Yoga Breath—Resting Position

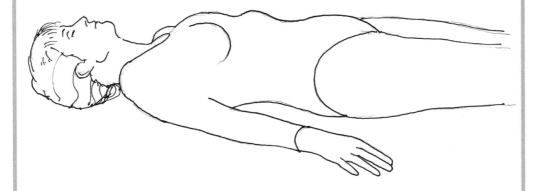

*To begin FYB, lie in a relaxed position on your back
and simply watch the rise and fall of the chest*

◆ *Inability to switch off/ sleeping problems*
◆ *Persistent infections*

Technique for Full Yoga Breath

Lie on the floor with your hands loosely beside your body, palms downward, and your feet flopped apart. Begin to watch your breath, and notice the following:

1. Does it feel as though your breath becomes stuck somewhere? For instance, it may become stuck around the middle of the abdomen or in the top of the chest.

2. Are your inhalations the same length as your exhalations?

3. Do you feel any strain on breathing in or out?

Stage 1

1. On your next breath, slowly inhale through your nose for the count of 4.

2. Expand your lower abdomen upward, feeling as though you are releasing a tight belt across your tummy. Feel the lower part of your lungs expand and fill with air.

3. Exhale for the count of 4, and consciously pull your abdomen muscles back down slowly, to flatten your stomach.

4. Repeat three times.

Focus: on the area around your belly button ballooning upwards with the inhalation and making sure all of your breath is exhaled, to empty your lungs and be ready for the next breath.

Stage 2

1. Inhale again slowly for the count of 4, and expand your lower abdomen.

2. Continue breathing for 2 more counts, and widen your ribs upward and sideways. Feel the middle part of your lungs fill with air.

3. Exhale for the count of 6, and allow your abdomen to flatten and the ribs to flatten also.

4. Repeat three times.

Focus: on the tiny muscles between each rib bone stretching, so your ribs can lift upward and sideways.

Full Yoga Breath—Stage 1

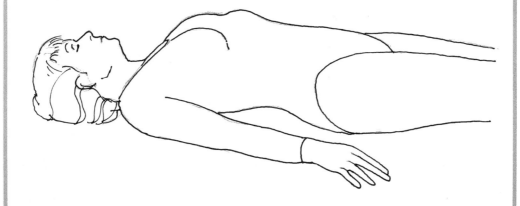

In Stage 1 of FYB focus on letting the abdomen balloon upwards on the inhalation and flatten on the exhalation.

Stage 3

1. Inhale slowly again, expanding your abdomen and ribs for a total count of 6.

2. Keep inhaling for another count of 1, and expand your upper chest muscles just under your collarbone. Feel the top part of your lungs fill with air.

3. Exhale for the count of 7, and feel first your abdomen, then your ribs and finally, the top of your chest empty of air. Repeat three times.

4. Combining all three stages, practice seven rounds of full yoga breath, inhaling and exhaling for a count of 7 each time.

5. Release the technique and return to the normal breathing pattern.

Focus: on the movement of your abdomen, ribs and upper chest being smooth and rhythmic, without strain, like the ebbing and flowing of a wave on the beach. Focus on a feeling of relaxation as you release the outward breath as slowly as possible.

Note:

♦ Remember that this is not a race, so do not rush the technique. Take time to become familiar with your breathing pattern, which is unique to each of us. With practice, this energy source and life force through the breath will become one of your most important tools for maximum health and well-being.

♦ Initially it's best to practice this breath lying down, until it becomes rhythmic and easy. Then it can be practiced standing or seated at various times throughout the day, to boost your oxygen and energy levels.

♦ The best time to practice this breath is when your body is relaxed, upon waking or the last thing at night before sleeping. For those who struggle out of bed each morning, try this breath seven times upon waking. As your body fills with oxygen and energizes your brain, your mind will become focused and it will be much easier to get out of bed. Use this breath at night if you cannot sleep, as the deep rhythmic pattern is very soothing to your mind before sleeping.

♦ At first, the technique may feel awkward. It takes time to undo bad breathing habits. Initially, exaggerate the movement of your chest to experience the full expansion and contraction of your lungs as they fill with air. The breath becomes quieter with practice.

♦ This deep, slow breathing technique is used when practicing many of the yoga postures; inhalations are used to gather energy within, and exhalations to extend and stretch into a posture.

♦ Do not be alarmed if you feel a little dizzy at the end of this breathing technique. When you practice this breath, simply make the count of 7 a little faster, until you feel comfortable. It takes time for the brain to become used to this increased amount of oxygen, especially if your breathing is normally shallow.

Full Yoga Breath—Stages 2 & 3

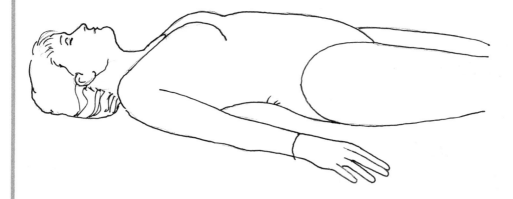

For stage 2 of FYB focus on allowing the ribs to lift upwards and sideways.
In Stage 3 allow the breath to fill the top of the chest.

Chapter **Three**

Routine One— Upper Body

(Approximately 20 minutes)

The five following chapters contain simple routines that you can practice at home without any special props or equipment. The purpose of the routines is twofold:

1. To build strength in the upper and lower body muscles for weight-bearing postures, which help the body to retain calcium in the bones. (Routines 1 and 2)
2. To improve the functioning of the endocrine glands, which contributes to strong healthy bones: the ovaries, adrenals, parathyroids, pituitary and pineal. (Routines 3, 4, and 5)

There is also a special chapter on yoga techniques to help alleviate menopause symptoms, including postures to improve the functioning of the glands that take over the production of estrogen-like substances at menopause: the pineal and adrenals. **(See the diagram in the introduction of where the glands are located.)**

STRUCTURE OF EACH ROUTINE

Each routine is structured so that when you are familiar with it, you can complete it in approximately 20 minutes. As your body strengthens, you can add more repetitions to each stretch or hold the postures for a longer time.

Each routine is divided into three sections: stretch, energize and breathe.

1. **Stretch:** Stretches build muscle strength, rotate the joints and improve the flexibility of the spine.
2. **Energize:** Weight-bearing postures build bone strength. Postures will energize and balance major endocrine glands and chakras in the body.
3. **Breathe:** Simple breathing techniques bring more oxygen into the lungs, which increases the metabolic rate and energy levels.

Each stretch, posture, and breathing technique includes the benefits and areas of focus to help you get the most from each one and to perfect it with practice. Visual images to keep in mind while practicing are provided for each of the yoga postures or asanas in the energize section. The yogis say that we are all energy beings, who transmit and receive energy from the environment and those around us. Energy is directed by thought. If you think that you are likely to be a possibility for osteoporosis because you have all of the indications, such as build, age or gender, then you will expect it to occur. However, with the very positive thoughts of hatha yoga, such as, "I am working on this; I am preventing this and building a stronger body," the energy follows the thought. You are then going to create what you believe in. Week by week, you will actually drench yourself positively with the knowledge that your body does not have to go downhill and degenerate. When the mind is given a very clear blueprint of the expected outcome from these routines, the energy will follow the thought and bring about the desired outcome. In other words, you must first see, in order to become the person you want to be.

ROUTINE ONE—UPPER BODY

This routine builds strength and flexibility in the upper body muscles and joints of the wrist, forearm, upper arm, shoulders, spine and neck. These are the areas where most osteoporosis fractures occur. Many women are weak in their upper bodies because of a lack of regular weight-bearing exercise. The old saying, "Use it or lose it" applies here. The more you use this routine, the more weight can be borne on your upper body, so that muscle strength is retained. In response to this weight-bearing stimulus, messages are sent to the body to retain calcium in the bones to keep them strong.

STRETCH

1. Wall Rotation

Benefits: This improves the flexibility of the spine and circulation to all·
the joints in the upper body to prevent stiffness and soreness.

Focus: on rotating your hips in both directions to a point of resistance,
to open up the spine. Do this stretch slowly and relax into the stretch.

1. Stand beside a wall with your left hip parallel to the wall and
   your hip just touching the wall. Your feet should be parallel to
   the wall and your arms extended along the wall in front, at
   shoulder height.

2. Inhale, walking your arms in a circle above your head while
   lengthening in your spine to lift your rib cage.

3. Exhale, and continue to walk your hands in a circle behind your
   back until they are at shoulder height. Look over your left
   shoulder.

4. Inhale, then exhale, and rotate your left hip and shoulder to the
   left. Move your right hip closer toward the wall.

5. Keep your feet parallel to the wall and slowly breathe in and out
   three times. On each exhalation, rotate your hips and shoulder a
   little more to the left, and walk your hands farther away from the
   body.

6. Return, by inhaling and walking your hands in a wide circle back
   over your head to the starting position.

7. Turn your right hip parallel to the wall, and repeat for three
   breaths on the other side.

Wall Rotation

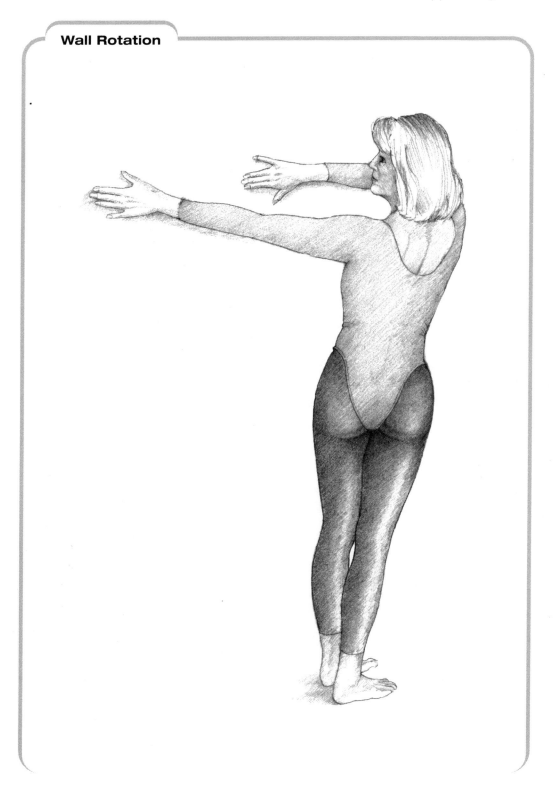

2. Balancing Tabletop

Benefits: This builds muscle tone in the upper arms, strengthens the wrist joint and stretches the hamstrings. It also releases tension all along the spine and builds bone strength as weight is borne for longer periods on the arms.

Focus: on moving your weight forward onto your hands to a point of resistance and then pushing your hips upward and backward to lengthen the spine.

1. Stand with your legs wide, feet turned out to the side, and your arms extended at shoulder height.

2. Bend forward, until your back is parallel to the floor, and hold this position for three breaths, while tightening your stomach muscles and keeping your legs straight.

3. Lower your outstretched arms to the floor. Have them shoulder-width apart and slide them back, so they are under your shoulders.

4. Lock your elbows and inhale. On the exhalation, move your body weight forward onto your arms, until your arms start to wobble. Keep your arms straight and hold for three slow breaths.

5. Keeping your hands on the floor, move your weight back into the heels and push the hips to the ceiling.

6. Push the head through the shoulders and push the weight into the back of your heels, keeping your hips high in the air.

7. Repeat three times.

Balancing Tabletop

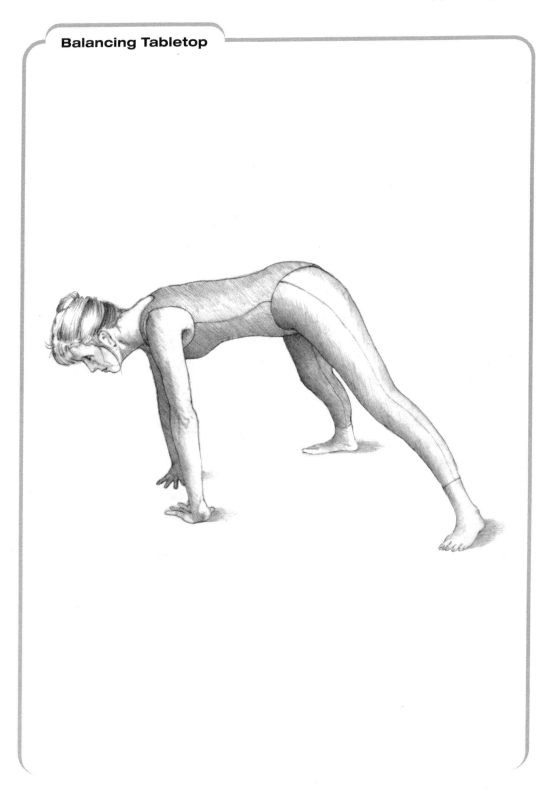

3. Downward-Facing Dog Posture

Benefits: This is a very strong position for building bone strength in the wrists, forearms and upper arms. Inverted positions also bring increased oxygen to the brain for clear thinking and release tension throughout the whole spine. This posture puts pressure on the pituitary gland situated deep in the brain behind the eyebrows, which is a super feedback system in the body that balances moods, appetites and sexuality among other things.

Focus: on the image of your body in a strong inverted "V."

1. Kneel on all fours, with your knees hip-width apart, and your toes tucked under. Spread your fingers apart.
2. Looking up, inhale and push your hips to the ceiling and straighten your legs.
3. Keep looking up, and push your weight into the back of your heels, while pushing up from the pads of your hands. Feel the stretch along your upper arms and along your armpits.
4. Drop your head through your shoulders and keep pushing your hips to the ceiling.
5. Work in the position by pushing up from the pads of your hands, and using the strength of your arms to push your head further through your shoulders.
6. Stretch your heels closer to the floor.
7. Hold this position for three breaths, kneel again, and rest.
8. Repeat again.

Downward-Facing Dog Posture

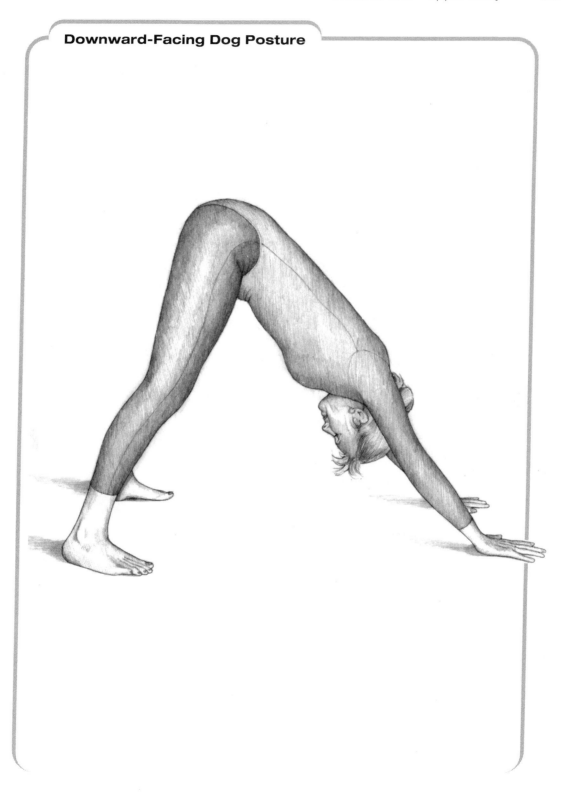

4. Extended Dog Posture

Benefits: This posture has the same benefits as the downward-facing dog posture, but with the added benefit of stretching the hamstrings.

Focus: on pushing up from the pads of your hands on the floor, while straightening both legs. Keep working your upper chest closer to your thighs by pushing your head through your shoulders.

1. Position your body on all fours with your heels against the wall.

2. Push into the downward-facing dog posture again, but this time take your right leg up the wall, turn your toes under, and straighten your right leg.

3. Use the strength in your arms to push your head through your shoulders, so your upper body comes closer to your thighs. Stretch through both legs.

4. Hold for 3 breaths.

5. To return, step your right leg down to the floor, bend your knees, and then sit back on your heels to rest.

6. Repeat, with your left leg extended up the wall, and hold for three breaths.

7. Release, by sitting back on your heels, and rest.

Extended Dog Posture

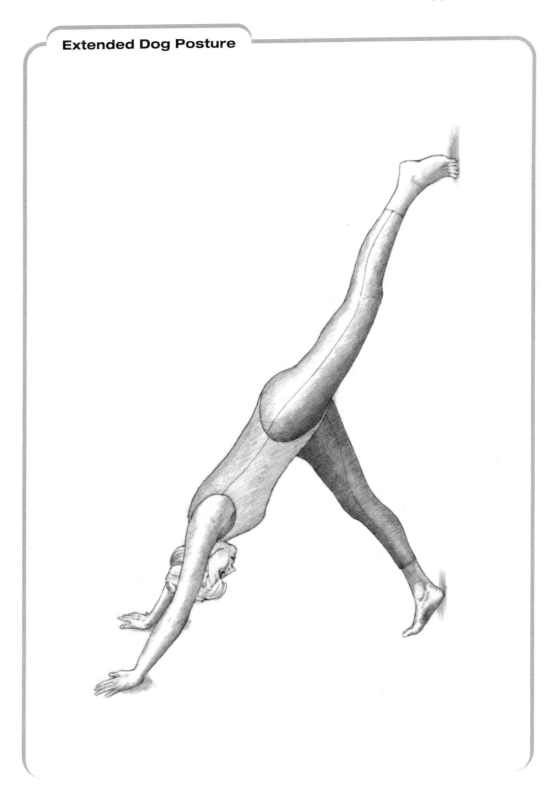

5. Dog Posture Reach

Benefits: This posture builds strength in the bones of the wrist, arm and shoulders, as weight is borne on this part of the body. Improves the flexibility of the hips and spine and releases tension throughout the shoulders.

Focus: on keeping your arms straight as you bend your knee to the three parts of your body, so your arms can support your body weight.

1. Move away from the wall and push into the downward-facing dog posture again on the floor.

2. Inhale, and stretch your right leg up into the air.

3. Exhale, and bend your right knee to touch your right wrist. Bend your left knee to the floor slightly in order to reach your right wrist. Hold for three breaths.

4. Inhale, and extend your right leg upward. Exhale, and, bending your right knee, touch your right elbow and hold for three breaths.

5. Inhale, and extend your right leg upward. Exhale, and bring your right knee to your forehead, while curling your back. Hold for three breaths.

6. Inhale, and stretch your right leg upward, and turn your hip slightly outward. Exhale, and hold the position for three breaths.

7. Inhale, and return your right leg to the floor, walk your hands back to your feet, and just hang loosely to regain your breath.

8. Repeat on the other side, holding each of the three positions for three breaths.

Dog Posture Reach

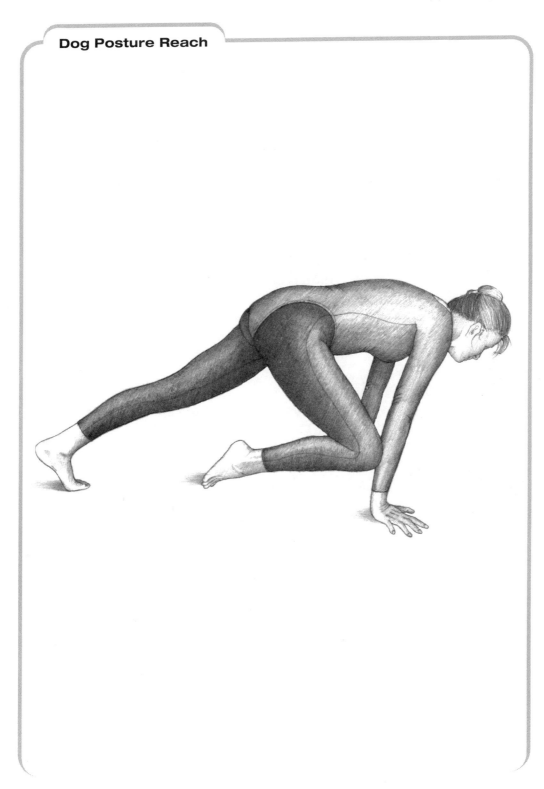

ENERGIZE

6. The Wedge

Benefits: This posture not only strengthens the bones of the wrists, arms and shoulders, but it stretches the solar plexus, the center of our emotional control. When negative thoughts and feelings dominate our lives, the solar plexus becomes very tense. This limits our emotional responses and breathing capacity. As the solar plexus is stretched in this posture, tension is released, the breath can flow more freely and emotional blockages are released. We can then express ourselves more clearly and do not waste needless emotional energy by constantly reacting and overreacting to life's situations. We become calmer, and more open and trusting in our relationships. The more clearly we can express our emotions, the less the people we live and work with need to be mind readers!

Focus: on a feeling of openness across your solar plexus and consciously letting your ribcage expand and contract easily with the breath. Imagine negative emotions flowing out with the breath, so that emotionally you have a clean slate to start each day.

Visualize: See yourself as a woman who is clearly able to express her emotions, and is valued for this openness. See yourself attracting other emotionally open people into your life who can uplift you.

1. Lie on your back with your feet flat on the floor on either side of your hips. Clasp your ankles firmly, pulling them close to your buttocks, and come up onto your toes.

2. Pinch your shoulder blades together and lift your hips to the ceiling, arching your back and moving your weight right into the back of your shoulder blades. Your chin is on your chest.

3. Place your palms behind the back of your waist with your fingertips pointing inward toward your spine.

4. Wriggle from shoulder to shoulder, and move your elbows closer together under your back to form a stronger arch.

5. Hold this position and breathe deeply in and out of your nose for seven breaths.

6. To return, slide your elbows out and lower your hips to the floor. Straighten your legs and rest with your arms loose by the side of your body, palms facing upward, and feet apart.

The Wedge

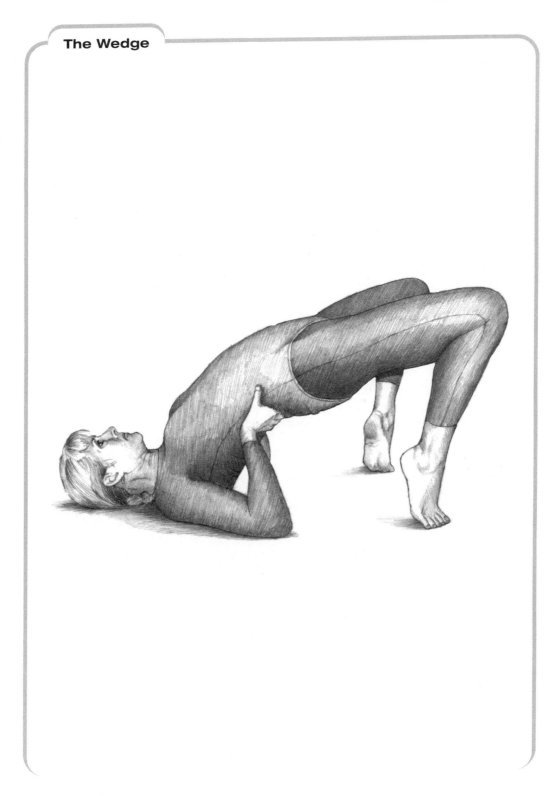

7. Cobra

Benefits: The cobra supports the weight of the body on the forearms and upper spine, to strengthen these bones. It also creates a lock over the thymus gland in the middle of the chest, which is responsible for our immune system. As the shoulder blades are squeezed together and the throat extended back, a lock is created over this gland in the middle of the chest, which restricts the circulation. As the posture is released, this part of the body is flushed with fresh, oxygenated blood to nourish and improve the functioning of the immune system. As we breathe deeply in the posture, more oxygen also reaches the heart muscle for better functioning.

Focus: on lengthening and stretching through your abdominal muscles, while arching upward and creating a strong lock from shoulder to shoulder and down the front of your throat, over the heart center.

Visualize: See yourself with a healthy immune system, free of disease. See your heart center opening, and your sense of compassion and forgiveness developing further.

1. Lie on your stomach with your forehead on the floor.

2. Bend your elbows and place your palms under your shoulders, with your forearms on the floor.

3. Inhale, and slide your chin and chest along the floor, while pushing on your hands, to arch your body upwards.

4. Lift your shoulders up, back, and down, away from your ears, squeezing your shoulder blades together. Arch your spine and push your chest out, while balancing on your hands. Keep your pelvis on the floor.

5. Drop your head back, and breathe slowly for three breaths.

6. To release, gently lower your abdomen, ribs and forehead to the floor, and return your arms loosely beside your body.

The Cobra

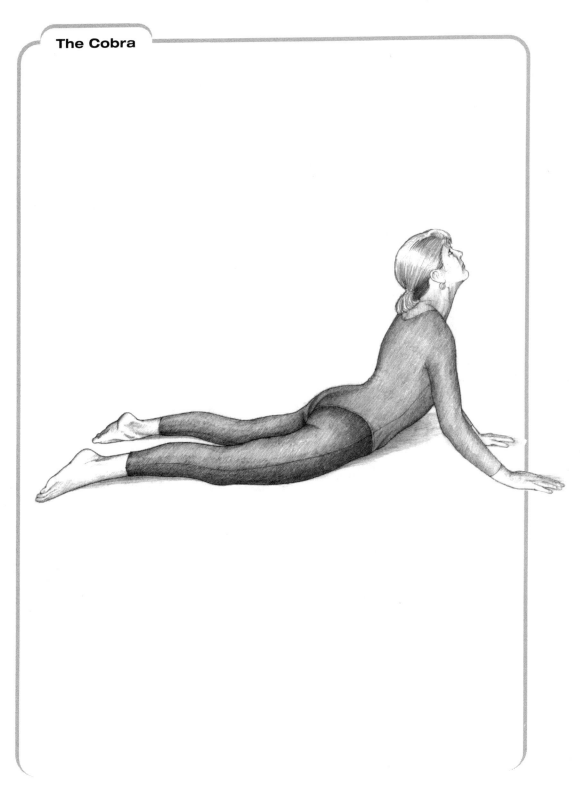

8. Balancing Crane

This posture should not be practiced by anyone with neck problems without the guidance of an experienced yoga instructor.

Benefits: This posture uses upper body strength to support the whole body on just the wrists, to strengthen these bones. As most women over 40 years of age weigh approximately 110 lbs.-plus, this is an excellent way to build strength in the upper arms and wrists. It also puts pressure on the pituitary gland in the head, which controls many hormone levels relating to our moods, sleep patterns, appetites, sexuality and intelligence. This posture allows fresh oxygenated blood to reach the head without the heart having to pump against gravity for clear thinking and improved focus. This posture is also excellent for improving your balance and concentration because if you don't concentrate, you fall on your head!

Focus: on keeping your weight evenly on both elbows, and tighten your tummy muscles to maintain balance.

Visualize: See yourself as a woman with strong arms, able to embrace all of life's situations. See yourself as perfectly balanced physically, emotionally and mentally, with a strong focus in life on all those projects that are so important to you.

1. Stand with your feet hip-width apart, and place your palms flat on the floor between your feet, with your fingers stretched wide.

2. Come up onto your toes, squat, and place your elbows firmly inside your knees.

3. Tilt your body weight forward and into your elbows, and then gently rock backward and forward, taking your weight onto your hands.

4. Repeat a couple of times, keeping your head down and your hips high, to be able to pivot your weight into your elbows. Adjust your hand position, if necessary.

5. With your weight forward into your hands, lift one foot off the floor, then the other, and balance on your elbows. Bring the soles of your feet together and breathe slowly three times. Tighten your stomach muscles to stay in balance.

6. Drop both feet back to the floor, and release.

Note: Practice this posture on a soft carpet, so that if you topple forward, the landing will be soft. This posture is actually easier than it looks, if the

Balancing Crane

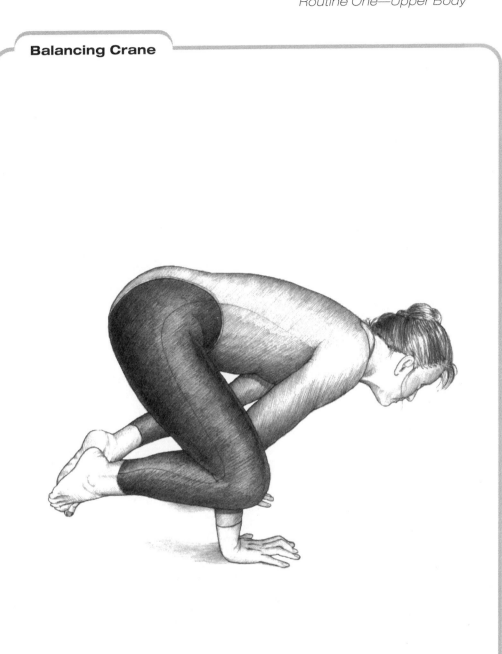

instructions are followed slowly and carefully, with concentration. At first you may only be able to hold this position for a few seconds, but as your strength and balance improve, you'll be able to hold it for longer periods of time.

BREATHE

9. Lung Stimulation Breath

Benefits: This breath is excellent for releasing tension and stiffness in the neck and shoulder area. It also strengthens the pectoral muscles in the top of the chest, to open up the upper part of the lungs and improve breathing capacity and oxygen levels in the blood. It is a very invigorating breath, which can also be used to release anger or frustration.

Focus: on pulling your arms back quite vigorously and keeping them at shoulder height, as you feel your pectoral muscles opening up and stretching.

1. Stand with your legs hip-width apart.
2. Have the palms of your hands on the front of your thighs.
3. Inhale, and lift your arms in front to shoulder height.
4. Clench your fists and, holding your breath, swing both arms out to your side at shoulder height and back to the middle again. Do not arch your back.
5. Still holding your breath, repeat six more times.
6. Exhale, open your hands, and release the palms back down to your thighs.
7. Repeat six more times.

Lung Stimulation Breath

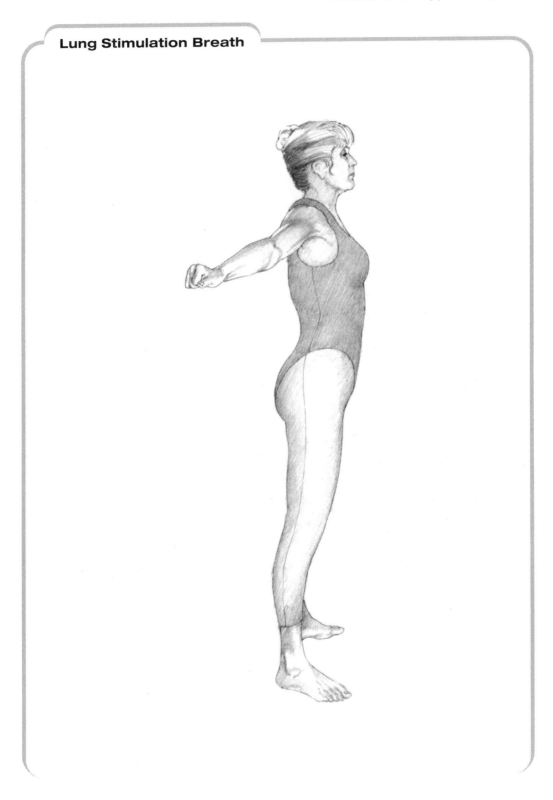

Chapter Four

Routine 2— Lower Body

(Approximately 20 minutes)

This routine builds strength and flexibility in the muscles and joints of the lower body, including the ankles, calves, thighs, knees and hip joints. This helps to maintain mobility throughout life. As the muscle strength improves, weight can then be borne on one leg at a time, to strengthen the bones of the lower body. Many people are strong in the legs, but often muscle-bound and inflexible because of repetitive-type exercises. The repetitive movements of many sports can shorten and tighten the muscles over time, leaving the body stiff and sore. Yoga stretches and postures lengthen the muscles and keep the joints flexible, so that over time, the body ages much better.

STRETCH

1. Bobs

Benefits: This stretches the inner thigh muscles and improves balance.
Focus: on keeping your back straight and pushing your knees wide on each squat.

1. Stand with your legs roughly hip-width apart, with your knees and toes turned out a little.

Bobs

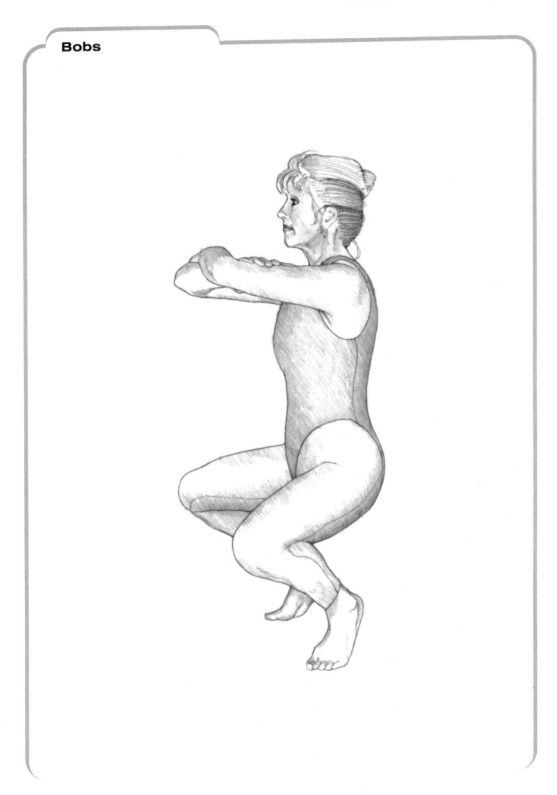

2. Clasp your elbows and, keeping your back straight and tummy tight, inhale, exhale, and squat.

3. Inhale, and return to the standing position.

4. Repeat 14 times, using the inhalation to straighten and the exhalation to squat.

2. Squats

Benefits: When the head is lower than the heart in this stretch, circulation to the brain is improved, for clearer thinking. The body does not have to push against gravity to move the blood to the brain. The weight of the head lengthens the muscles around the vertebrae, so that the spine can release trapped muscles and nerves, and both circulation and energy to this area improve.

Focus: on feeling the stretch from your hamstrings, right through to the whole of your spine, as you straighten your legs.

1. Stand with your legs hip-width apart, lean forward and place your clenched fists on the floor inside your feet. Squat down, keeping your fists inside your feet, and your elbows inside your knees.

2. Straighten your legs, pushing the hips high to the ceiling, but keep your fists firmly on the floor. Drop your head down. Feel the stretch in your hamstrings.

3. Repeat this squat and straightening of the thighs seven times.

Squats

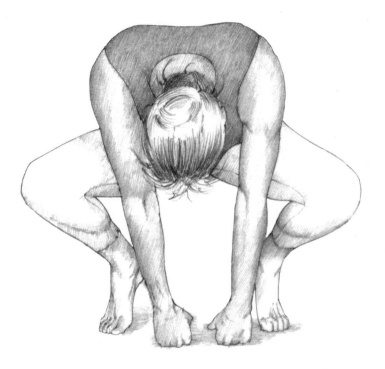

3. Squat and Rock

Benefits: This improves the strength and flexibility of the upper thighs and hip joint, as well as balance.

Focus: on keeping your balance and stretching your inner thighs by pushing your knees out with your elbows.

1. Stand with your legs wider apart, with your toes and knees turned out. Clasp your elbows.

2. Inhale, and straighten your back. Exhale, and squat slowly, keeping your balance. Hold your breath for a few seconds.

3. Inhale, and straighten your legs to the original standing position.

4. Repeat seven times, using the inhalation to straighten and the exhalation to squat.

5. Next, squat and place the palms of your hands together in front of your chest and wedge your elbows inside your knees.

6. Rock from side to side seven times, pushing your elbows into your knees each time.

7. To release, place your hands on the floor, straighten your knees, and stretch your hips up to the ceiling.

8. Repeat again if you can, then release by placing your palms on the floor and straighten your legs, letting your head hang loosely.

Squat and Rock

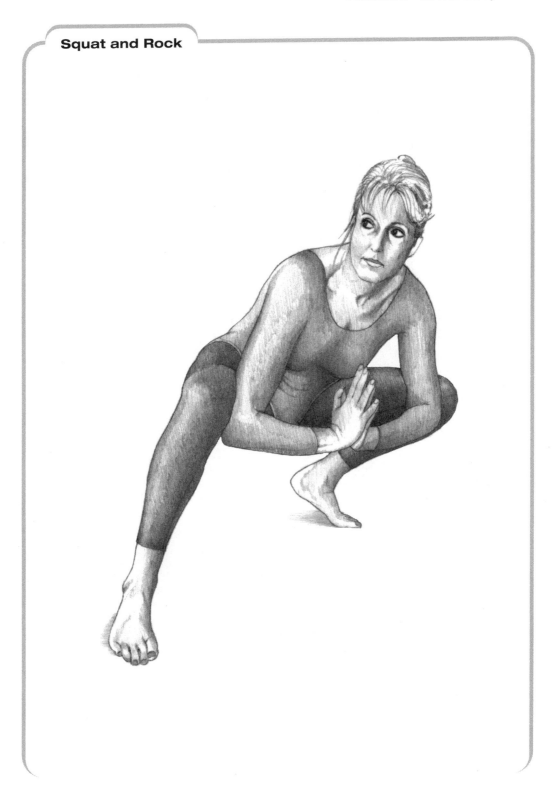

4. Lunges

Benefits: Lunges stretch and strengthen the upper thigh muscles and improve balance.

Focus: on keeping your hips facing forward and keeping your upper body upright.

1. Stand with your legs wide apart and arms stretched out to shoulder height.

2. Turn your right foot out to the side and look to the right.

3. Inhale, and level your hips, so they face forward. Exhale, and lunge to the right as low as possible. Keep your hips to the front, and back upright. Inhale, and return.

4. Repeat two more times. Turn your right foot in and your left foot out, looking to the left side.

5. Repeat three times on the other side.

Lunges

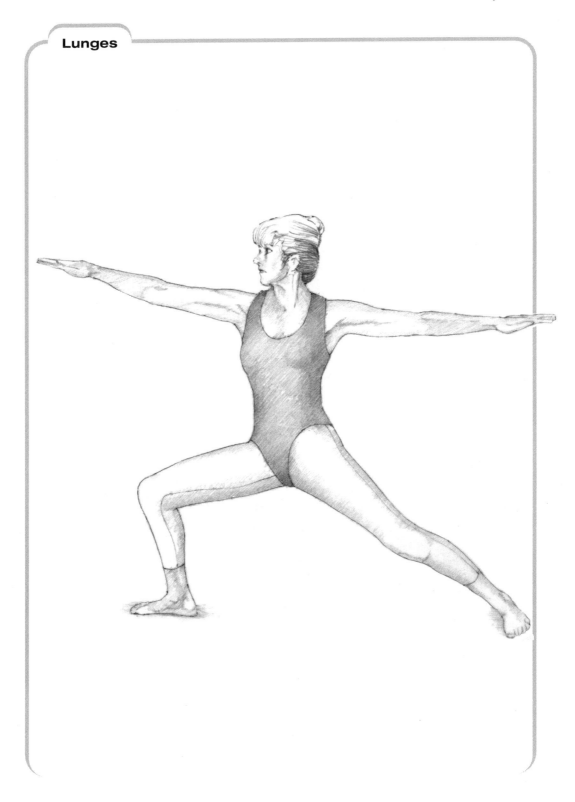

5. Standing Extended Lunge

Benefits: This rotates the hip and shoulder joints to a point of resistance, to improve circulation and flexibility. It also releases tension in the neck and shoulders and strengthens the upper thigh and calf muscles.

Focus: on pulling your shoulder and hip back strongly, and look up under your arm each time.

1. Stand with your legs wide apart and your right foot turned out. Your arms are stretched out at shoulder height. Look to the right.

2. Inhale, and stretch up through your spine. Exhale, bend your right knee, and lunge to the right.

3. Place your right palm on the floor, inside your foot.

4. Bring your left arm over your head, palm downward, until your arm is flat against your ears

5. Breathe evenly for four breaths. On each exhalation, rotate your left hip and shoulder back, and lengthen through your left arm and fingers of your left hand.

6. Lunge low enough to feel your upper thigh muscles stretch.

7. Inhale, and return. Repeat two more times on this side, then change sides and repeat three times to the left side.

Standing Extended Lunge

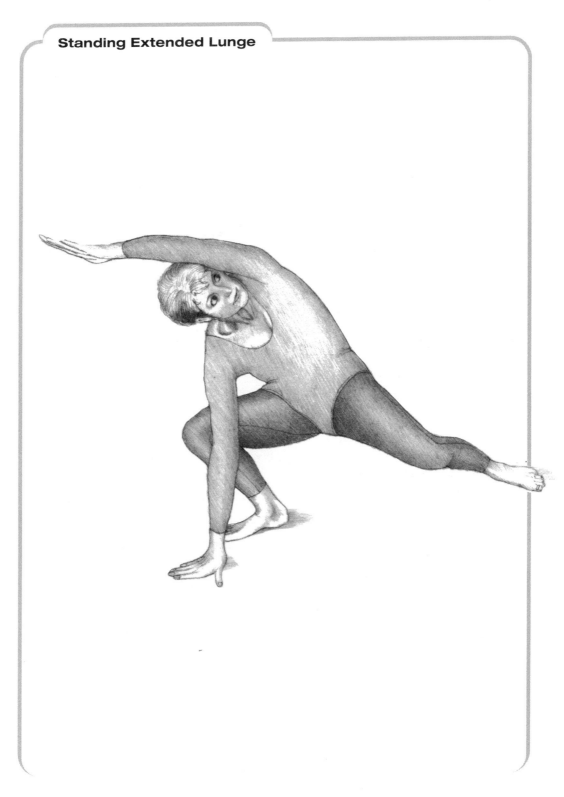

6. Feather and Tipple

Benefits: This is a wonderful stretch for the spine to improve flexibility. It also strengthens the bones and joints of the wrists and ankles, as they support the body's weight.

Focus: on lengthening through the front of your body and thighs, so your hips can lift a little higher off your buttocks to improve the stretch.

1. Sit on the floor with your heels drawn into the groin. Clasp your feet and draw your heels as close to the groin as possible, with your elbows inside your knees.

2. Keeping your hands firmly on your feet, bounce your knees up and down to the floor seven times, to stretch your inner thigh muscles.

3. Make two fists and place them behind your buttocks. Inhale, take your weight on your fists, and lift your hips.

4. Exhale, part your feet, and come onto your toes. Push your hips upward and arch your back, while stretching your knees to the floor.

5. Drop your head back, pinch your shoulder blades together, and lift your buttocks off your heels.

6. Breathe slowly seven times as you hold this position, stretching through the front of your thighs, and at the same time, feeling a strong stretch through your emotional center near your solar plexus.

7. To return, take your weight on your fists, lift your knees off the floor, and draw them in close to your chest.

8. Repeat again, taking your knees to the floor, and breathe slowly seven times.

9. To release, sit back on the floor and straighten your legs.

Note: If you cannot take both knees to the floor, try stretching one at a time to the floor. In time, your thigh muscles will lengthen and stretch.

Feather and Tipple

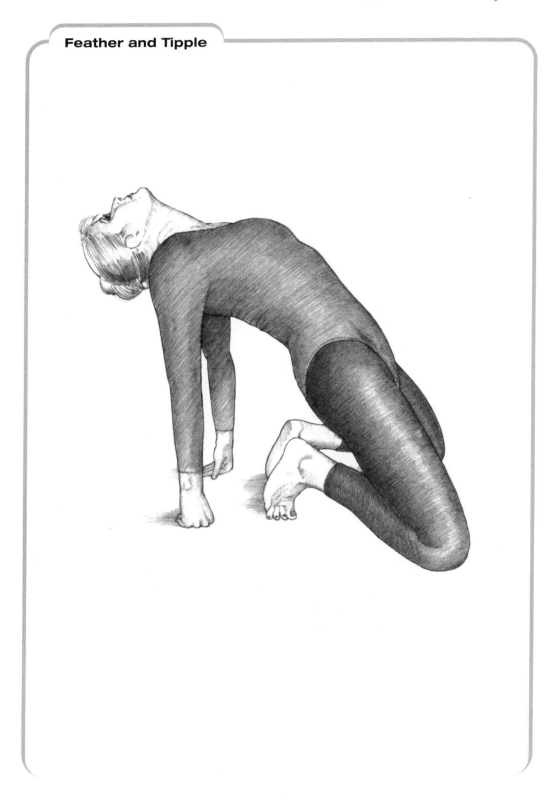

ENERGIZE

7. Pose of a Dancer

Benefits: This is a calming yet strong posture, where the entire body weight is borne on one leg at a time to build bone strength and improve balance, concentration and coordination, which are important in preventing falls as we age.

Focus: on creating a strong arch in your lower back to put pressure on the adrenal glands, which control stress levels. To do this, pull your foot up, back, and away from your buttocks slowly to improve the position.

Visualization: See yourself as steady, calm and graceful in this posture.

1. Stand with your legs hip-width apart, and bend your right knee. Take hold of your right foot with your right hand, and balance on your left leg.

2. Lock your left leg strongly and push up from the floor with your left foot.

3. Inhale, and lift your right foot back, up, and away from your buttocks.

4. Exhale, and at the same time, stretch your left arm out in front of you and hold the balance.

5. Breathe slowly three times, and then lower your right leg to the floor.

6. Change sides, and hold the balance for three breaths on the other side.

Pose of a Dancer

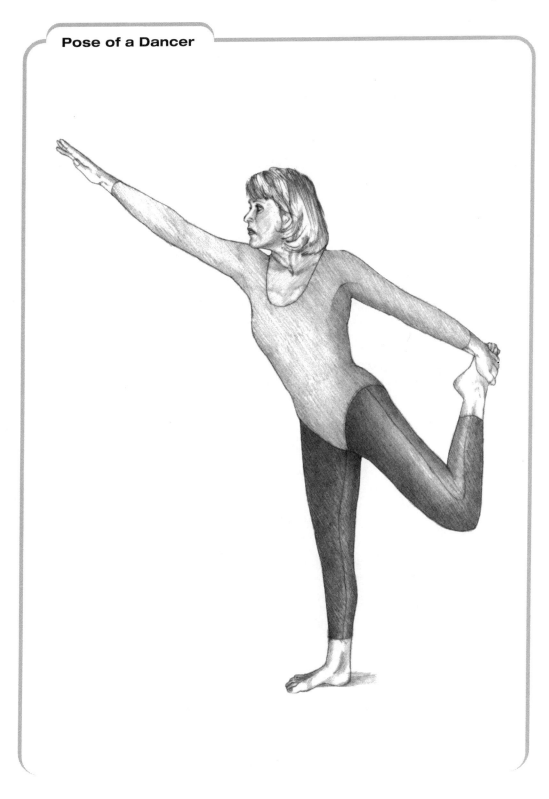

8. Balancing Spine Twist

Benefits: This strong posture is designed to rotate the hip, shoulder and neck joint to a point of resistance, to increase circulation and prevent stiffness and soreness. It also builds bone strength in each leg and the wrists, while improving balance.

Focus: on keeping your supporting leg locked and straight for support, and your palm flat on the floor. Aim to flatten as much of your body against the wall as possible as your hips and shoulders are rotated.

Visualization: See your spine as flexible and free of tension, so there is space between each vertebra for the energy to flow freely. See the messages from your central nervous system flowing freely between your body and your brain without obstruction, so that you think more quickly, and react faster to life's opportunities.

1. Stand with your back against a wall, with your legs wide apart and your arms stretched out to shoulder height.

2. Turn your right foot out and look to the right.

3. Inhale, and lengthen through your spine. Exhale, and lunge to the right, placing your right palm on the floor, about a foot in front of your right foot. Lean into the wall with your hip for support.

4. Inhale, and straighten your right leg. Exhale, and lift your left leg parallel to the floor, against the wall.

5. Inhale, turn, look up, and extend your left arm up to the ceiling.

6. Exhale, and rotate your left hip and shoulder flat against the wall.

7. Hold the position for three breaths, as you work to flatten as much of your body against the wall as you can.

8. To return, lower your left leg to the floor, and come back into the standing position.

9. Turn your right foot in and left foot out and repeat to the other side, holding your balance for three breaths.

Balancing Spine Twist

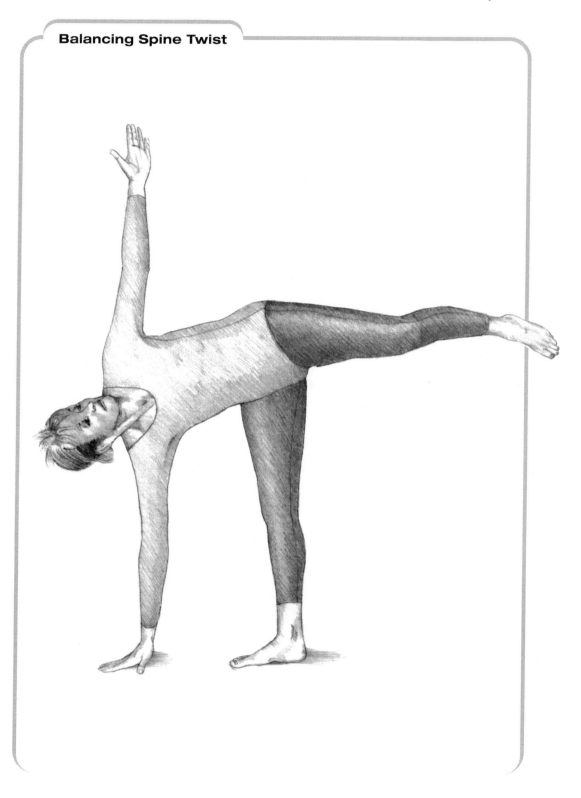

9. Pose of a Warrior

This position can be practiced freestanding, or with the help of a chair in the early stages.

Benefits: This is an empowering and energetic balancing posture to strengthen each leg, improve balance, and stretch the shoulder and hip joints to release any stiffness and soreness.

Focus: on keeping your standing leg locked, to prevent wobbling and stretching horizontally in a straight line from hands to hips to feet, once in the position.

Visualize: See yourself as a powerful woman with the confidence to stand alone when need be, as symbolized by standing on one leg at a time.

1. Stand with your legs wide apart and clasp your hands over your head with the first finger of each hand touching, like a steeple. Turn your right foot out.

2. Inhale, and stretch up through your spine. Exhale, rotate your body to the right, and lunge onto your right foot, keeping your arms stretched upward.

3. Look up at your hands, and pull your shoulders back. Push your hips forward, and balance for three breaths.

4. Lean forward, and take your arms level with the floor, while straightening your right leg.

5. Take your weight on your locked right leg, and slowly lift your left leg up, until it is parallel to the floor.

6. Stretch out through your left hip joint, by lengthening through your left leg.

7. Pick something to focus on to hold your balance and breathe slowly for three breaths.

8. To return, lower your left leg to the floor, returning to the lunge position, and bring your hands over your head again, with shoulders back.

9. Straighten your right leg, and rotate your body back to the starting position.

10. Turn your right foot in, your left foot out, and repeat to the other side.

Note: Initially, you can use a chair to support your outstretched arms, and when balanced, practice lifting your arms off the chair for an increasing length of time, until you can practice freestanding.

Pose of a Warrior

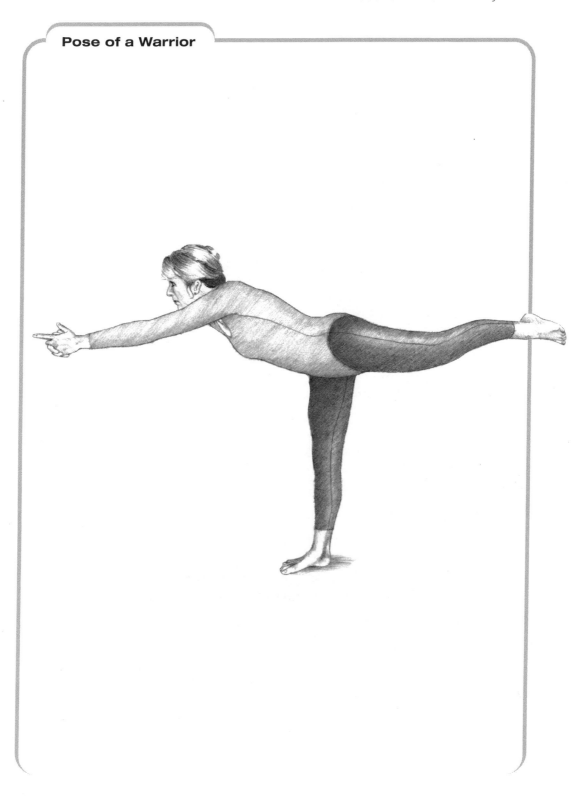

BREATHE

10. The Etheric Breath

Benefits: This breath is a very conscious way of working with the body's power to heal itself, and is an excellent breath to practice directing energy to parts of the body that need to be strengthened or repaired. We each have the ability to heal both ourselves and others. We only need to create the right conditions for healing to occur, and consciously direct energy and thoughts to assist this healing process. This breath can also be used to direct energy to someone who needs healing, and if enough people around the world send energy to that same person at the same time, it can become a very powerful force for healing.

Focus: on mentally charging this energy from your breath with the energy from each of the three centers: heart, solar plexus, and spleen. See the part of your body you choose being flooded with charged energy, to heal, repair, and strengthen it. Know that energy always follows thought, and if the thoughts are of a healing nature, then the directed energy will also be of the same nature.

1. Sit cross-legged on the floor, or with your legs outstretched, or seated.

2. Inhale slowly through your nose, and imagine that you are drawing golden energy down through the crown of your head to the heart center.

3. Hold your breath, and mentally move this energy around from your heart to your solar plexus, to your spleen (the spleen is on the left side of the body, under the heart), and back to your heart in a triangle shape three times.

4. As you exhale, mentally direct your energy to a part of your body that needs to be strengthened or healed.

5. Repeat for six more breaths, either directing the charged energy to the same part of your body or to a different part each time.

6. To release, go back to your normal breathing technique, and sit quietly for a few moments, visualizing the damaged area being healed, or another person being healed.

Note: You do not have to believe in this technique for it to work; just try it for yourself, and see what happens over time.

The Etheric Breath

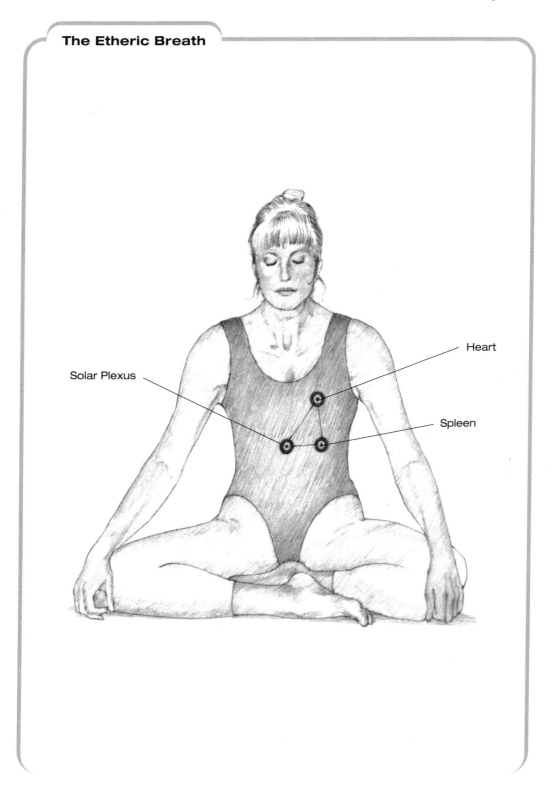

Chapter Five

Routine 3— The Ovaries

(Approximately 20 minutes)

This routine builds strength and flexibility in the spine, by releasing trapped nerves, improving circulation and energy levels. This improves communication levels between the brain and the body via the central nervous system. The health of the spine is integral to the overall well-being of the body, and the yogis say that a flexible spine means a flexible mind. The flexibility of the spine is crucial to being able to practice the forward-bending postures, which create a strong lock and pressure over the ovaries to promote the balanced flow of estrogen and progesterone for regular cycles.

STRETCH

1. Spine Stretch

Benefits: This stretch releases trapped energy along the spine and rotates the shoulder joint, to increase the circulation to this area and release stiffness.

Focus: on lifting up through your rib cage and lengthening along your spine with each inhalation.

1. Stand with your legs hip-width apart, and clasp your hands in front of you.

Spine Stretch

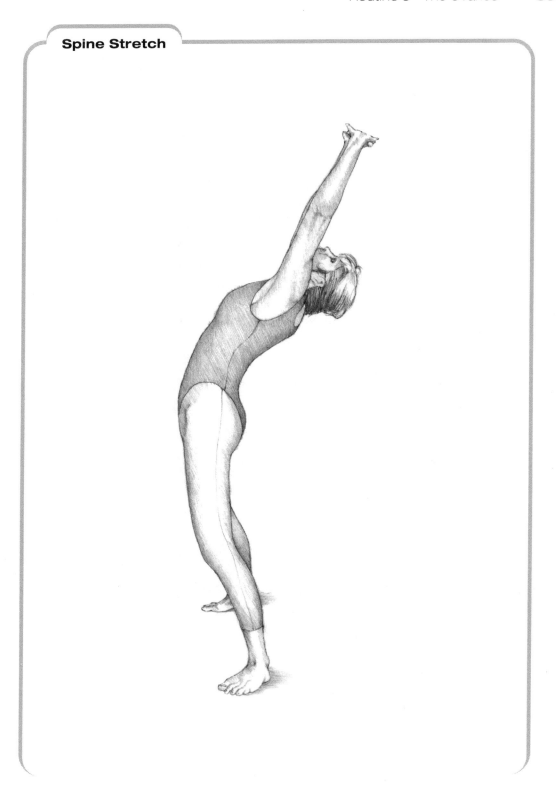

2. Inhale, and push your hands away from you, palms outward, as you lift your hands up and over your head.

3. Lift up through your abdomen, and stretch your arms back through your ears.

4. Lock your legs, hold this position for a few seconds, and arch backward.

5. Open your arms wide, and exhale, returning your arms to the starting position, with hands clasped.

6. Without taking a breath between each stretch, repeat seven times.

2. Side Spine Stretch

Benefits: This stretches the muscles at the side of the waist, shoulders, neck, and hips, for increased flexibility.

Focus: on pushing each hip outward strongly, with your legs locked, and leaning into the posture as far as you can. Do not be surprised if you hear a few noises with this posture as your spine realigns itself with the stretches.

1. Stand with your feet apart, and your hands clasped above your head. Invert your hands, so your palms are pushing upward, towards the ceiling.

2. Inhale, and lengthen through your spine.

3. Exhale, and lean over to the right side, while pushing the left hip outwards and stretch the arms away from the body. Aim to keep the body in a flat plane.

4. Inhale back to the center. Exhale, and lean over to the left side.

5. Repeat, doing six stretches on each side.

Side Spine Stretch

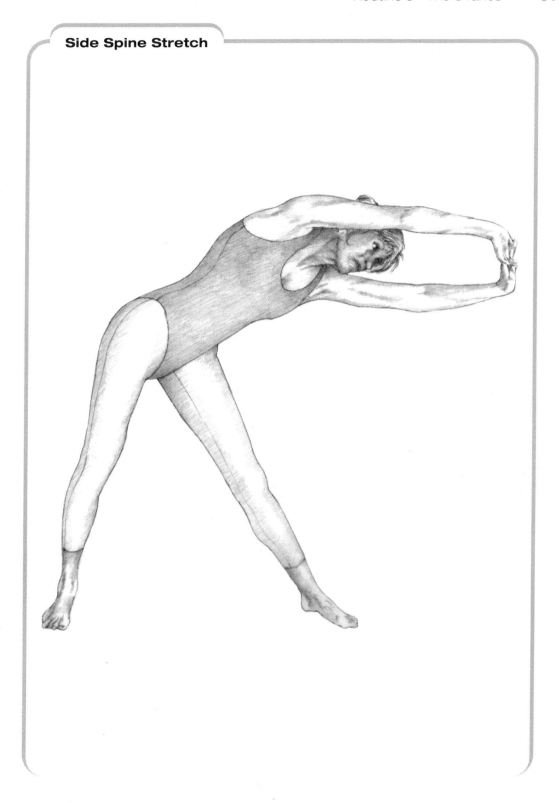

3. Backward Arch

Benefits: This strong stretch opens up the spine and strengthens the upper thigh muscles. It also puts pressure on the adrenal glands in the small of the back that control our stress levels and take over the production of estrogen-like substances at menopause.

Focus: on keeping your knees bent slightly when taking your weight backward and pushing firmly into your feet, to maintain balance.

1. Stand with your legs wide apart, and your knees slightly bent.

2. Place your hands behind your waist, with your fingers pointing in toward your spine.

3. Inhale, and stretch through your spine. Exhale, bend your knees slightly, and lean backward, taking your weight evenly on your thighs.

4. Push your hips forward, pinch your shoulder blades together, and let your head hang between your shoulder blades.

5. Inhale, and return to the starting position.

6. Exhale, and bend forward, until your back is level with the floor, keeping your hands on your waist.

7. Lock your legs firmly, and arch your back, stretching through your hips.

8. Inhale back to the starting position.

9. Repeat this arching and bending forward slowly seven times, using the inhalation to bring your body back to the center each time.

Backward Arch

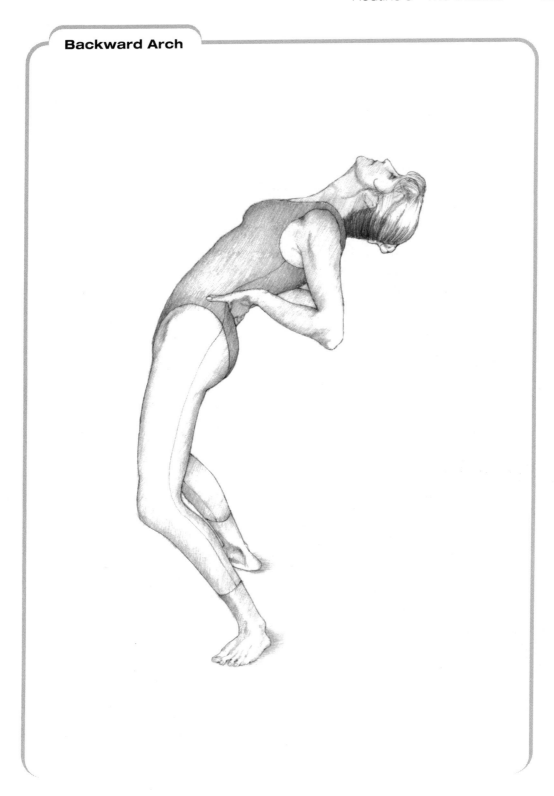

4. Cat Stretch

Benefits: This is a favorite posture of many students, to release tension throughout the whole spine. It keeps the spinal and shoulder muscles strong and flexible, while releasing tension in the neck and shoulders. It also strengthens the tummy muscles, which support the spine to prevent back problems later in life.

Focus: on sucking up your stomach muscles really hard under your rib cage, and on pushing up under your shoulder blades.

1. Kneel on all fours on the floor.

2. Inhale, and suck your tummy in hard, while rounding your back and dropping your head through your shoulders. Feel as though you are pushing something off the back of your shoulders.

3. Exhale, and arch your spine, pushing your chin forward and your buttocks out.

4. Repeat this arching and rounding seven times.

Cat Stretch

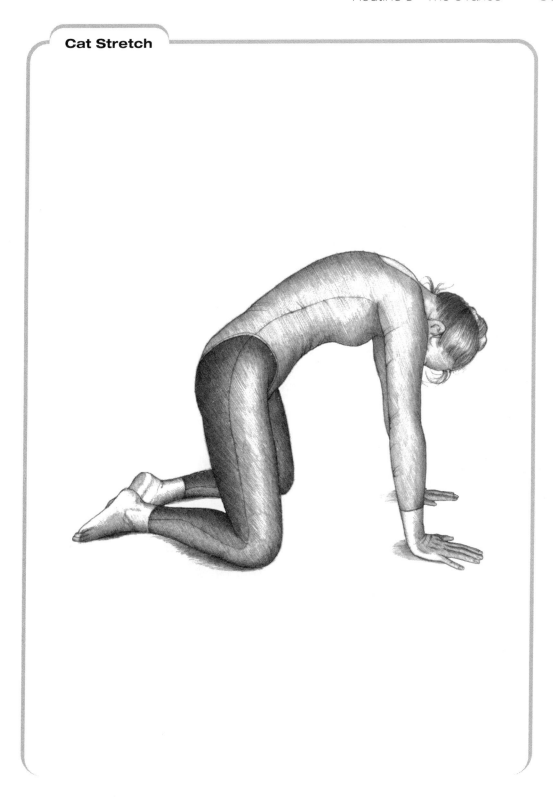

5. Kneeling Side Stretch

Benefits: This is a good strong stretch all along each side of the body, with the added benefit of rotating the shoulder and hip joint to a point of resistance for increased flexibility. It increases circulation and flexibility to the neck, shoulder and hip joint. It also improves flexibility of the whole spine, and improves wrist strength for weight-bearing exercises

Focus: on lengthening through each side of your body with each sideways stretch, and on rotating your hips and shoulder back to a point of resistance.

1. Kneel on the floor, with your left knee bent and your right leg extended out to the side, with your toes pointed to the floor. Extend your arms to shoulder height.

2. Inhale and lengthen through the spine.

3. Exhale, and lean over to the left, placing your left palm on the floor to the outside of your knee.

4. Bring your right arm over and lay it close to your ears, keeping your arm straight and palm downward.

5. Inhale, and lengthen through the right side of your body.

6. Exhale, and while looking up, rotate your right hip and shoulder back, to open the joints.

7. Inhale, and return to the center. Then exhale, and slide your right hand down your right leg, as far as possible.

8. Bring your left arm over your head and lay it close to your ears, with your elbow straight and palm downward.

9. Inhale, and lengthen through the left side of your body.

10. Exhale, and looking up, rotate your left hip and shoulder backward, to open the joint.

11. Return to the center, and repeat two more times on each side, using the inhalation to lengthen, and the exhalation to rotate the joint.

12. Change sides, and kneel, with your right knee bent and your left leg extended. Repeat three times on each side.

Kneeling Side Stretch

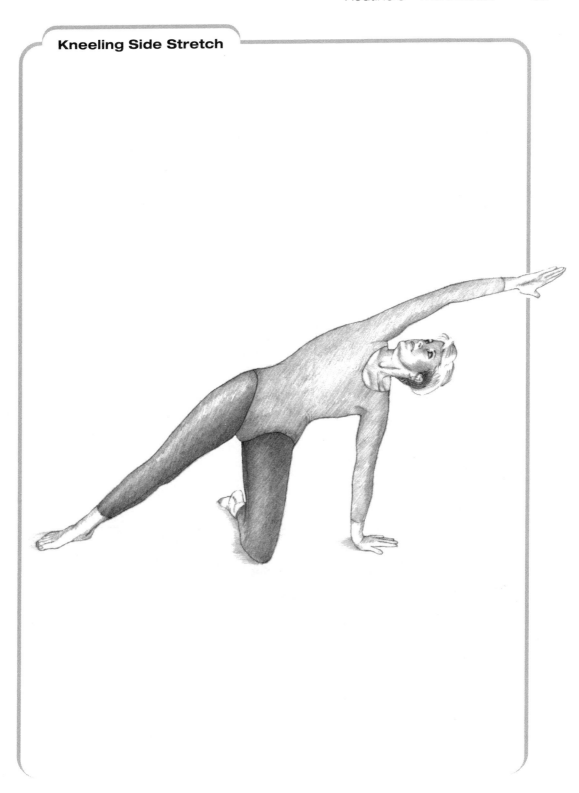

ENERGIZE

6. Seated Spine Twist

Benefits: This seated posture releases trapped nerves and frees up the energy throughout the spine. It rotates the hip and shoulder to a point of resistance, to open up the joints. It also stretches the hip muscles, to prevent stiffness and soreness.

Focus: on stretching up through your spine on the inhalation, and softening and rotating your hip and shoulders on the exhalation. Do not force your body to twist, but gently ease into the position, using the breath.

Visualization: Visualize your spine as strong, flexible and free of any stiffness, soreness or pain. See yourself as being flexible, and able to handle change in your life. Visualize yourself as open to new ideas, people and opportunities.

1. Sit on the floor with your legs extended in front of you.
2. Bend your right knee, and step your right foot over your left leg
3. Bend your left knee, and curl it under your right knee, making sure you sit evenly on both buttocks.
4. Place your hands with fingers turned inward at either side of the hips.
5. Turn to the left, inhale, and extend your left arm to shoulder height.
6. Exhale, and hook your left arm tightly around your right knee, pulling it in close to your body.
7. Turn to the right. Inhale, and extend your right arm to shoulder height.
8. Exhale, and place the back of your hand behind the small of your back.
9. Inhale, and lift up through your rib cage, to lengthen your spine.
10. Exhale, and looking to the right, pull your right shoulder and hip back.
11. Breathe three times, each time rotating your hip and shoulder back on the exhalation.
12. Untwist your body, take a slow breath, and repeat on the other side.

Creative Power Postures

These postures work on improving the health and functioning of the ovaries. They use the flexibility in the spine to extend along the front of the body, creating a lock over the reproductive glands. This pressure over the glands restricts the circulation to the area temporarily, and when the posture is

Seated Spine Twist

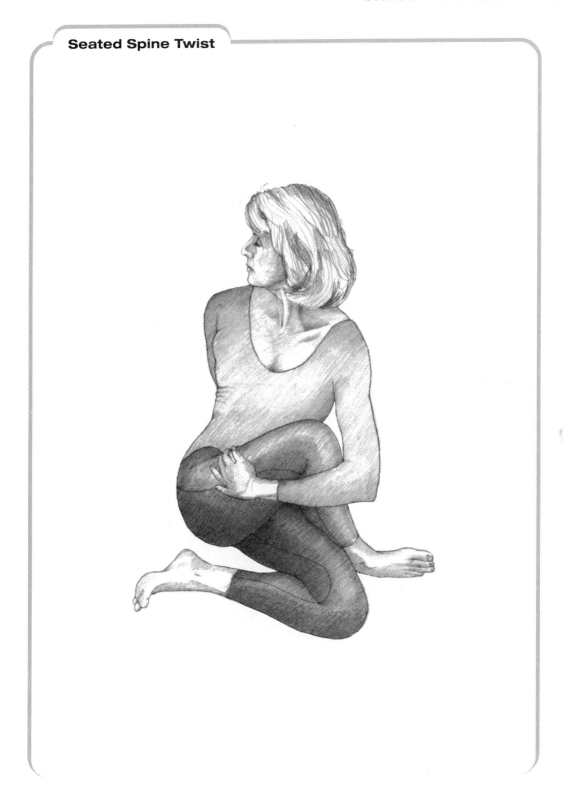

released, this area is flooded with fresh, oxygenated blood, to nourish these glands that produce estrogen and progesterone. Unfortunately, studies have shown that long before the onset of menopause, a good proportion of women age 30 and younger fail to ovulate each month. This can sometimes result in a progesterone deficiency. Normally, when an egg is released during ovulation, the follicle enlarges and changes to become the corpus luteum. This secretes progesterone, so that if the egg is fertilized, it can implant successfully. However, when a woman fails to ovulate regularly, as in the case of some female athletes, there is no corpus luteum formed, and a progesterone deficiency can occur. Studies show that bone-making cells have progesterone receptors for making new bone. A lack of progesterone can lead to less bone tissue being made and thinning of the bones, making them more prone to the onset of osteoporosis.

A number of yoga postures work on improving the health and functioning of the ovaries. Regular practitioners of yoga state that yoga reduces the intensity of PMS symptoms, from which an estimated 40% to 60% of all women suffer. Regular students of yoga also report that their monthly cycles become more regular, the more they practice yoga postures. More regular cycles increase the likelihood that estrogen and progesterone levels will be balanced, with better chances of maintaining bone density.

7. Bent Leg Creative Power Posture

Benefits: This posture improves functioning of the ovaries, which produce and reproduce every cell in your body. If these glands are healthy and function as they should, sloughing off the old cells and making the new cells, you will not age prematurely. It also strengthens the lower back muscles and stretches the hamstrings.

Focus: on creating a strong lock over your groin, while lengthening in the back of your spine. Also focus on breathing deeply and consciously sending energy to your ovaries, to nourish them.

Visualization: In each of the following Creative Power Posture variations, see your ovaries being flushed free of toxins, with increased blood flow to this area. See them behaving as they should, sloughing off the old dead cells of the body, and creating new cells, so that you do not age prematurely. See your monthly cycles being in balance, so that PMT and menopausal complaints become less disruptive to your life. Visualize your creativity being released, because according to yoga philosophy, the health of the ovaries contributes to your creative energy, as well as your reproductive energy.

1. Sit on the floor, with both legs extended in front of you.

2. Bend your right knee, and place your right heel close beside the outside of your right buttock.

Bent Leg Creative Power Posture

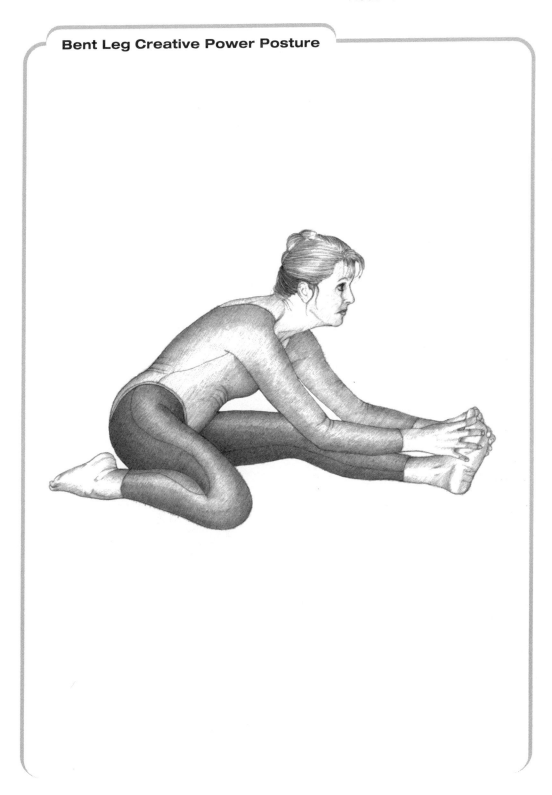

3. Place both hands, fingers turned inward, at either side of your hips.

4. Inhale, and stretch your arms above your head, lifting up through your rib cage, to lengthen through each side of your spine.

5. Stretch out of your right side, then your left, twice through each side.

6. Keeping the length in your spine, exhale, bend forward, and clasp your left ankle.

7. Inhale, and lengthen in the front of your chest, and push your chin forward.

8. Exhale, and bend your elbows, bringing your chest closer to the top of your thighs.

9. Keep looking up at your toes, and focus on creating a lock over your groin, to limit the circulation to your ovaries. Lengthen in the back of your spine.

10. Hold this position, as you breathe slowly for three breaths, each time lengthening in the front of your body, and squeezing into your groin on the exhalation.

11. To release, stretch your hands forward and above your head in a wide circle, and return to the start.

12. Straighten your right leg, and bend your left knee close into your left buttock, and repeat on the other side, holding the position for three breaths.

8. Standing Creative Power Posture

This is quite a strong position and takes time to master so be patient.

Benefits: This posture improves the functioning of the ovaries and increases the circulation to the head, for clear thinking, as the head is inverted to the knees. It really stretches the hamstrings and the lower back very strongly.

Focus: on sliding your buttocks up the wall and bringing your head closer to your knees, to improve the lock over your ovaries with each exhalation.

1. Stand with your back against a wall, with your feet hip-width apart.

2. Inhale, stretch your arms over your head, and then stretch and lengthen out of both the right and left side of your body, while lifting up through your spine.

3. Bend forward with a flat back, and clasp your ankles. Drop your head down, as close to your knees as possible.

Standing Creative Power Posture

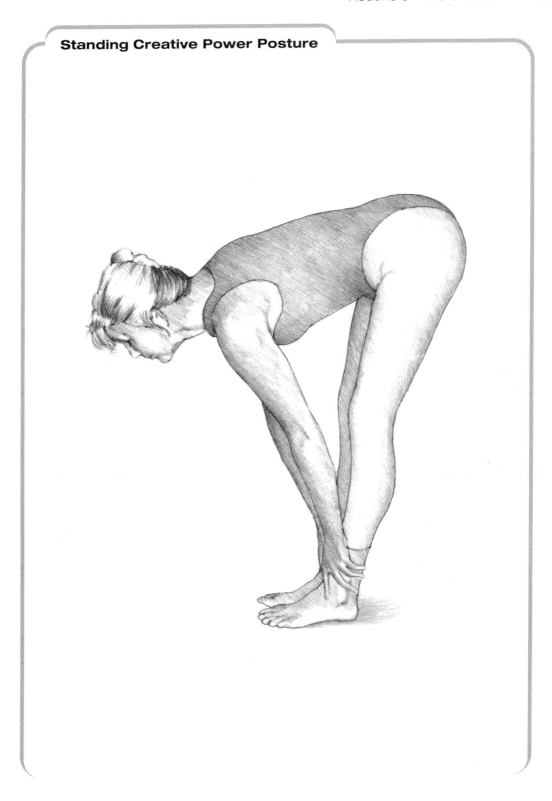

4. Holding onto your ankles, inhale, and stretch your chin forward, lengthening in your spine.

5. Exhale, bend your elbows, and draw your chest down along your upper thighs, creating a lock over your ovaries.

6. Using the breath, inhale, and stretch away with your chin.

7. Exhale, and squeeze your upper body closer to your groin, while pushing your buttocks higher up the wall, to improve the lock.

8. Repeat the stretching and squeezing for five more breaths.

9. To release, stretch your hands forward above your head, and take them in a wide circle back to your thighs.

BREATHE

9. Tibetan Breath

Benefits: This breathing technique opens up the upper chest muscles, to improve breathing capacity. It also releases tension throughout the spine and shoulders.

Focus: on pulling your shoulder blades back strongly at the end of each inhalation, and on keeping your movements smooth and rhythmic.

1. Stand with your feet hip-width apart and your arms loosely beside your body.

2. Bring your fingertips together over the front of your hips.

3. Look to the right, and inhale, moving your weight into your right foot.

4. Stretch your right arm up toward the ceiling, and extend your left arm upward at the same time, while you count from 1 to 7.

5. Look up at the fingers of your right hand, pull your shoulders back, and open up your chest. Hold for three counts.

6. Exhale for the count of 7, while you lower your arms to the starting position, with fingertips touching.

7. Look to the left, move your weight into your left foot, and repeat on this side.

8. Repeat seven times on each side.

9. Note: If you run out of breath before the end of seven counts, take one more smaller breath, pull your shoulders back, and continue to lift your arms.

Tibetan Breath

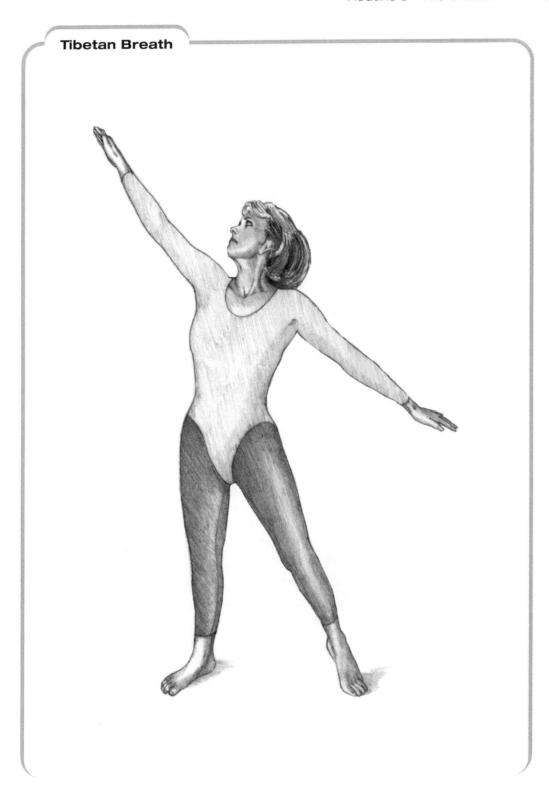

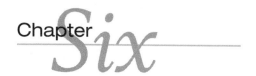

Routine 4— The Adrenals

(Approximately 20 minutes)

This routine builds flexibility in the hip joint, to prevent falls and fractures as we age. The hip muscles and joints are deep inside the body, and are difficult areas to access. The following stretches deeply rotate the hip to a point of resistance, to free up the joints, so that the muscles can stretch and strengthen. As breathing is deepened, there is an increased supply of oxygen and blood flow to the joint, to nourish, repair and regenerate the cells of this part of the body.

Flexibility and strength are also needed in the hip joint, in order to practice the back-bending postures that create a lock over the adrenal glands, to regulate stress levels in the body. More manageable stress levels lead to less excretion of calcium from the body and stronger bones.

STRETCH

1. Hip Rolls

Benefits: This stretch rotates the spine, hip, and shoulder area, to release stiffness and soreness in the joints and improve flexibility. It is especially good, first thing in the morning, for an easy stretch to release lower back stiffness.
Focus: on bringing your knees up to your elbow, and not vice versa.

Hip Rolls

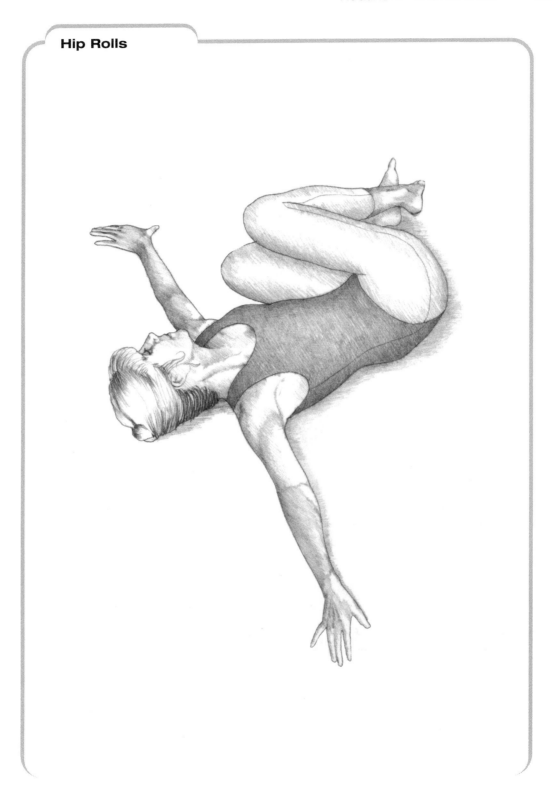

1. Lie on the floor, with your knees bent to your chest. Stretch your arms out on the floor at shoulder height, with your palms down.

2. Inhale, then exhale, and roll both of your knees over to meet your right elbow. Look to the left, and push your left shoulder down.

3. Inhale, and take your knees back to the center. Then exhale, and push both of your knees to your left elbow, while looking to the right.

4. Push your right shoulder down.

5. Repeat seven more times on each side.

2. Cross-legged Hip Roll

Benefits: This is a full rotation of the hip and shoulders to a point of resistance, to improve flexibility and circulation to these joints.

Focus: on keeping your shoulder down, and bringing both of your knees as close to the floor as possible.

1. Lie on the floor, cross your right knee over your left, and tuck your right foot behind your left ankle. Place your left foot back on the floor.

2. Keeping your foot on the floor, inhale, and draw your left foot in close to your buttocks.

3. Exhale, and drop both knees to the left on the floor, while rotating your hip. Look to the right, and push your right shoulder into the floor.

4. Hold this position, and take three slow breaths. On each exhalation, push your right shoulder into the floor.

5. Inhale, and return your knees to the center. Then repeat to the same side two more times.

6. Return your knees to the center, cross your legs the other way, and repeat three times to the right side.

Cross-legged Hip Roll

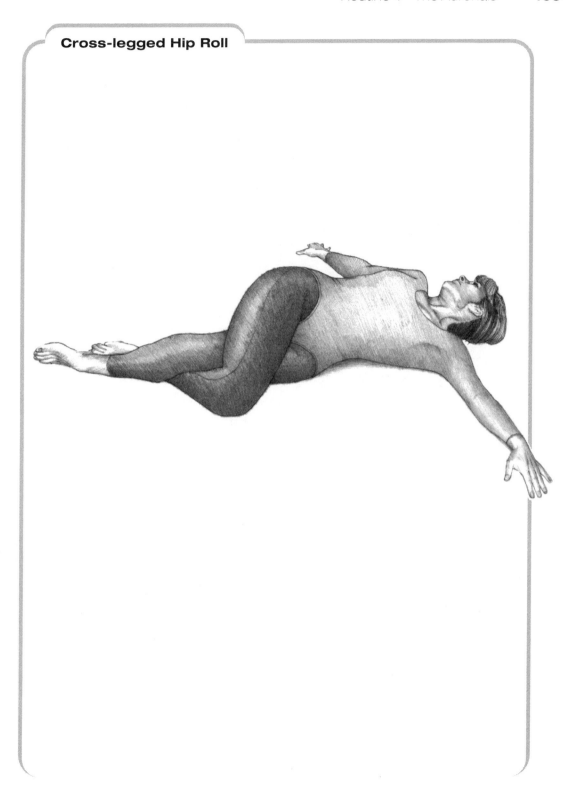

3. Crossed-Ankle Stretch

Benefits: This opens up the hip joint, stretches the lower back, and improves flexibility of the hip joint.

Focus: on lengthening in your lower back, and on stretching your hands away from your body with each exhalation.

1. Sit on the floor with your legs outstretched, place your right ankle over your left, and bend your knees slightly. Pull out your buttocks from beneath you, so that your hips are firmly on the floor.

2. Inhale, and stretch your arms above your head, stretching out of the left and right side a couple of times, and lift up out of your rib cage.

3. Exhale, and, keeping the length in your spine, bend forward and place both hands, palms down on either side of your crossed ankles.

4. Inhale, and stretch your chin forward.

5. Exhale, and lower your head between your knees, feeling a deep stretch in your hip joint. Let your knees relax outward.

6. Take three slow breaths. Stretch through your lower back, and walk your hands on the floor, farther away with each exhalation.

7. Keep your head low, between your knees.

8. To release, inhale, and stretch your hands above your head. Then exhale, and return them in a wide circle to the sides of your body.

9. Cross your ankles the other way, and repeat on the other side for three deep breaths.

Crossed-Ankle Stretch

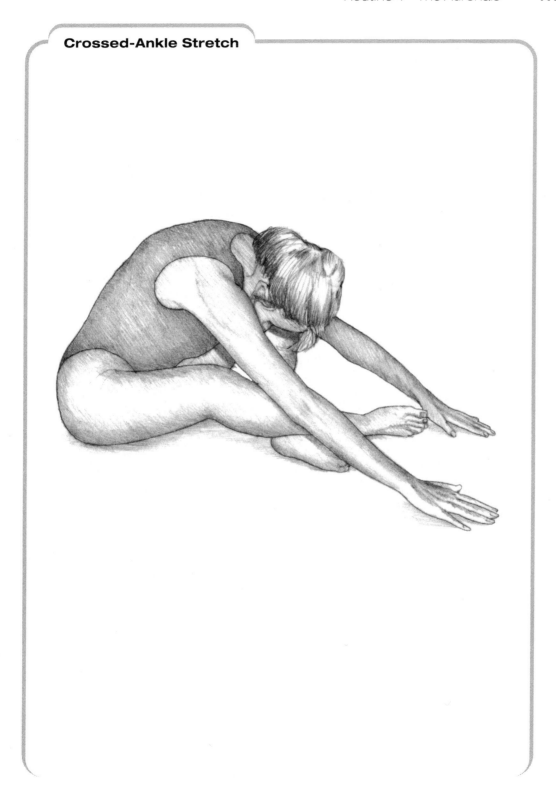

4. Deep Hip Stretch

Benefits: This deep hip stretch really gets into the tight parts of the hip joint and stretches both of the large buttock muscles, to release stiffness and tightness. If you want a greater challenge in this position, wiggle both feet outward, away from the body, while in the crossed position. The feet should be level across the front of the body. Then rest the chin on the knees.

Focus: on giving in to the deep stretch in the hips rather than fighting it.

1. Kneel on all fours, and cross your left knee in front of your right.
2. Wiggle your right foot away from your body, to make space to sit back in between your heels, with your weight evenly on both buttocks.
3. Place your hands, one on top of the other, on your knees.
4. Inhale, and lengthen along your spine.
5. Exhale, and place your forehead or chin on your knee. Relax your elbows around your knees.
6. Hold that position, and breathe deeply three times, relaxing your shoulders and letting all of your weight come down evenly through both buttock muscles.
7. Release, by lifting your forehead or chin off your knees.
8. Rock your body forward, and place both palms on the floor. Bring yourself back onto all fours again.
9. Untwist your legs, and cross your right knee in front of your left. Repeat on the other side for three breaths.

Deep Hip Stretch

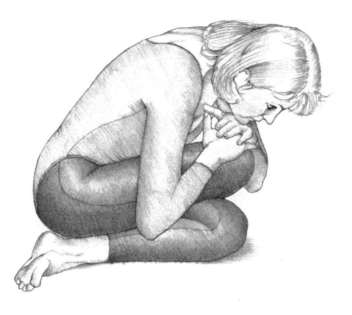

5. Pose of a Child

Benefits: This posture keeps the hip joint open, while resting between yoga postures. It allows the spine to be softly stretched and the upper thighs to be stretched.

Focus: on flattening your body to the floor, as much as possible, and on keeping your hips down.

1. Kneel on all fours on the floor, lean back, and take hold of your calf muscles.

2. Roll them outward, and sit deeply between your hips, with your buttocks touching the floor.

3. Place your arms loosely beside your hips, with palms facing upward.

4. Keeping your buttocks on the floor for as long as possible, stretch your chin forward, and gently lower your forehead to the floor.

5. Initially, your buttocks will lift upward, but once your forehead is on the floor, keep pushing them down to further stretch your spine.

6. Round your back, let your shoulders drop closer to the floor, and relax into the position in a very passive way.

ENERGIZE

These postures use the flexibility of the hips to create a lock over the adrenal glands, which sit on top of the kidneys. These glands control our stress levels. Prolonged stress in our lives leads to depletion of calcium levels and thinning bones.

The adrenals also produce estrogen-like substances during menopause that can offset declining estrogen levels from the ovaries. However, for this to occur, the adrenals must be in good shape. Unfortunately, many working women, whether in or out of the home, enter menopause with depleted adrenal glands. This is often caused by stressful lifestyles and lack of attention to a program of sound nutrition and exercise.

Some of the negative stress experienced by women today is often caused by feelings that they are not utilizing their full creative potential. For example, they may be stuck in boring, repetitive jobs, like the routine running of a house, playing chauffeur to children all day, or boring, repetitive office jobs. These frustrating and stressful feelings can increase the adrenaline levels in the body, causing a state of "red alert" in which the person feels constantly anxious and ready for action. Without a constructive outlet for this anxiety, emotional exhaustion can result and long-term, chronic tiredness and fatigue can lead to depletion of calcium levels.

Pose of a Child

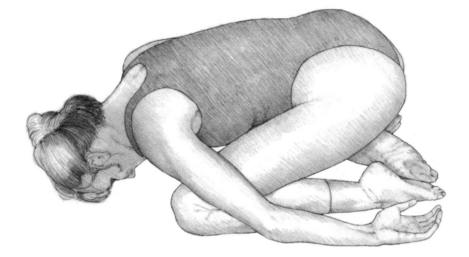

A further problem arises from the interrelationship between irregular cycles and stress. Stress, combined with a bad diet, can induce irregular menstrual cycles and lower progesterone levels, which can have adverse effects on bone density. As progesterone is a building block for the hormones that protect us against stress, this lack of progesterone interferes with the production of these stress-combating hormones. This exacerbates stress, gives rise to further irregular menstrual cycles, and so the vicious circle continues.

A number of yoga postures help to break this cycle, by bringing the adrenal glands back into balance. It is the hormones produced by the adrenal glands that give us our fight-or-flight mechanism and our ability to succeed in life. When they are out of balance, tension and stress are the result. This stress can be positive or negative. Positive stress can come from the tension caused by the will to create, which uses energy positively, such used on an all-absorbing creative project. You may be working under stress, but it is pleasant stress. Negative stress can be compulsory, and is often bought about by fear or anxiety. This can be caused by being in a position above your capabilities, and pushed to produce more than you can realistically achieve. It is this negative stress that yoga works to relieve through balancing the adrenals, so that general anxiety levels are more manageable. When this happens, a person can more realistically assess where the stress is coming from and the cost, health-wise.

6. Bow in Cat Posture

Benefits: This posture creates a strong lock over the glands that control our stress levels, and limits the circulation to this area. As the posture is released, the glands are flushed with fresh oxygenated blood, to keep them functioning in a balanced way, maintaining manageable stress levels. This posture also works on a deeper level on the chakra relating to our will power, and on strengthening it. The longer a person can hold this position, the more the will power improves.

Focus: on pulling your foot away from your buttock (not toward it) to create a stronger lock in your lower back.

Visualize: When we are stressed, we behave more aggressively. This posture releases stress, so visualize aggression levels falling, while assertiveness is enhanced. As it also works on the will power, visualize your will power strengthening, and know that you can keep going long after you think you can't.

1. Kneel on all fours, with your palms down, and lock your right elbow.

2. Bend your right knee, and reach around with your left hand and take hold of your right foot.

3. Holding your balance steady, inhale, and lift your foot up, back and

Bow in Cat Posture

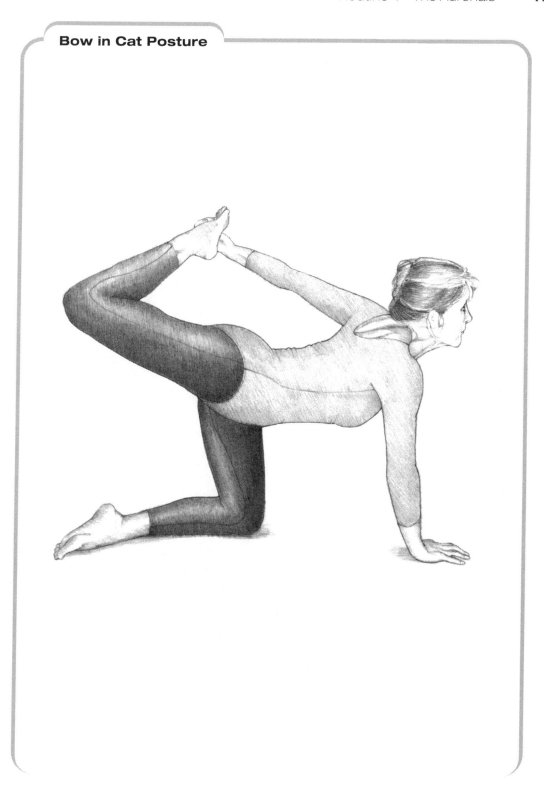

away from your buttocks, to create a lock in your lower back over the adrenal glands.

4. Breathe slowly, and keep lifting your foot and knee high, to create a greater lock.

5. Keep your right elbow locked, for support, and look up.

6. Hold this position for four breaths, and on each exhalation, lift your knee a little higher.

7. Release your knee and hand to the floor, and arch and round your back two or three times, to release the lock in your back.

8. Lock your left elbow, bend your left knee, and reach around with your right hand to grasp your left foot. Repeat on the other side, and hold the position for four breaths.

7. Camel

Benefits: This is one of the most liberating and empowering positions I know of for women. The solar plexus, or emotional center, is free of tension, which calms the nerves. The spine is open, to free up the flow of energy to and from the central nervous system, for clear thinking. A lock is created over the adrenal glands, to help regulate the stress levels.

Focus: on keeping your hips arched and your weight moving forward into your knees. Imagine breathing out negative emotions with your breath, to clear emotional blockages and recharge the solar plexus.

Visualize: As this posture opens up the emotional center, freeing it of negative energy, see yourself as an unlimited storehouse of loving energy available to yourself and others.

1. Kneel on the floor with knees apart and feet flat. Lift the buttocks off the heels and rest the palms on the front of the thighs. The front of your feet should be flat on the floor.

2. Inhale, stretch your right arm above your head, and arch backward.

3. Exhale, and grasp hold of your right heel firmly, while locking your elbow.

4. Drop your head back.

5. Inhale, and stretch your left arm up above your head. Exhale, and grasp your left heel firmly.

6. Pinch your shoulder blades together, and push your hips forward.

Camel

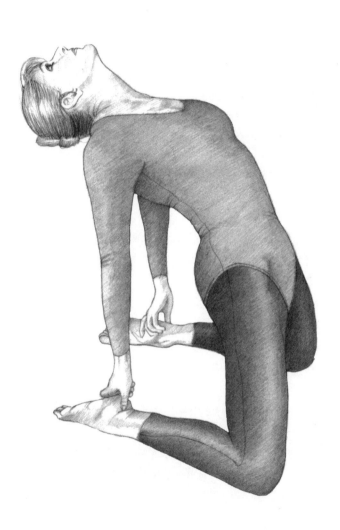

7. Push your weight forward into your knees, arch your spine, and breathe slowly and deeply seven times.

8. To return, keep your head back, bend your elbows, bend at the waist, and lower your hips between your heels again.

9. Drop your head to the floor in the Pose of a Child, and rest.

10. Repeat on the other side, starting with your left arm first.

8. The Swallow

Benefits: This beautiful, liberating and strong position supports all of the body weight on the pelvic area. It also creates a strong lock over the adrenals, while improving the strength and flexibility of the spine.

Focus: on lifting your body off the floor into a strong "V" position.

Visualize: See yourself able to fly like a bird, as symbolized in this posture, and achieving your greatest goals and aspirations in this lifetime.

1. Lie on the floor with both arms stretched out in front, and your forehead on the floor.

2. Inhale, and then exhale, lifting just your thighs off the floor.

3. Hold the lift, while breathing slowly for three breaths, and then lower your thighs.

4. Inhale again, and then exhale, lifting your head and shoulders off the floor, stretching your arms out strongly in front.

5. Hold steady for three breaths, lifting your arms a little higher with each exhalation, and then return your upper body to the floor.

6. Inhale, and then exhale. Lift both your thighs and your upper body off the floor at the same time.

7. Swing your arms back, and pinch your shoulder blades together.

8. Balance on your pelvic area, feeling as free as a bird, and breathe deeply three times.

9. Release the position, and rest on the floor.

Fall Prevention

The regular practice of these weight-bearing yoga postures to strengthen the hip joint and bones will help prevent falls and fractures throughout life. While white women have a 17% lifetime risk of hip fracture, this figure appears to be lower in other ethnic groups. The average age for someone

Swallow

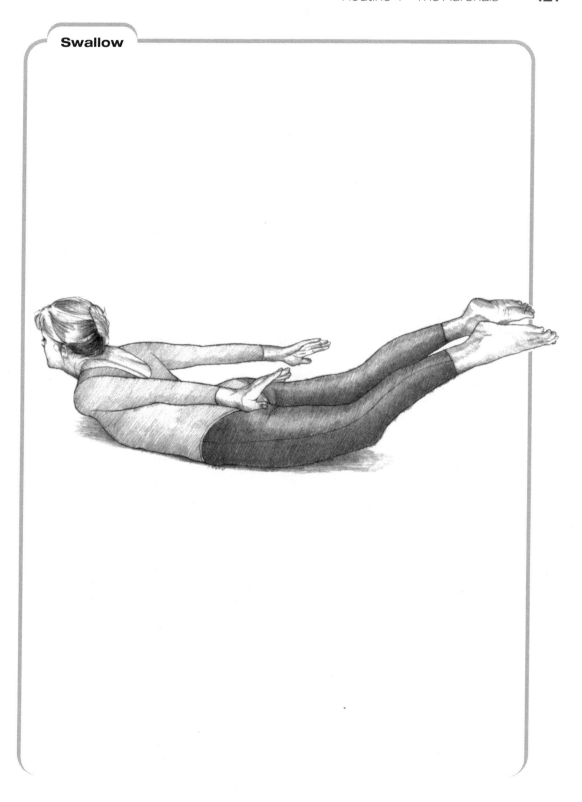

Forward and Backward Falls

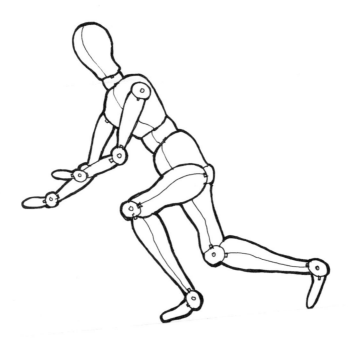

*A forward fall will be broken by the arms
which will protect the hips*

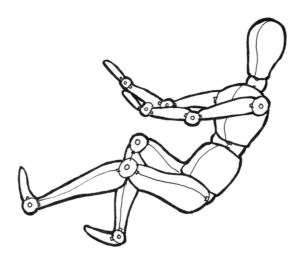

*A backward fall is borne directly by the hips
and increases the risk of a hip fracture*

experiencing a hip fracture is around 80 years. Many of these occur in nursing homes, where the use of barbiturates is high and disorientation occurs. It is difficult to determine whether a person falls first and then breaks a hip, or the hip breaks first, and then the fall occurs.

When muscle strength, balance and coordination skills are maintained well as we age, a fall need not necessarily result in a serious fracture. If the pace of walking is sufficiently brisk, then a fall will be forward, onto the extended arms, breaking the fall and protecting the hips.

When muscle strength, balance and coordination are impaired, a fall will be backward, directly onto the hip, without the protection of the arms breaking the fall.

Most osteoporosis fractures occur in the upper body, and can vary from serious to mild discomfort, but a hip fracture can create serious, life-threatening complications. Within 90 days of a hip fracture, 10% to 15% of patients will die, due to complications, while 20% will die within the first year. Approximately 50% will never regain the quality of life they had before. Therefore, it is critical for women who are over 40 years old to practice these sorts of weight-bearing postures regularly, in order to build strength and flexibility in the hips and avoid the risk of a hip fracture later in life.

BREATHE

This technique helps to correct the problem of erratic breathing, which often occurs during times of stress. Erratic breathing causes sighing and lifting of the shoulders, and the lungs never fully empty between breaths. This makes taking another breath difficult, and, combined with a feeling of not being able to get enough air, creates anxiety and panic. Throughout the day, the shoulder and neck muscles tense from continually lifting the shoulders, as breathing becomes more difficult. This can cause a vicious circle of hyperventilation, more tension, and greater anxiety.

Benefits: This technique can be used to manage a panic or anxiety attack, as it reduces excess air in the lungs. Deep, rhythmic breathing is also very soothing to the mind, and in time, will lower the feelings of anxiety, as the breath returns to normal.

Focus: Visualize letting go of all the air in your body, in order to make space in your lungs for the next inhalation. Imagine that all the busy thoughts in your mind are flowing out with your breath. Imagine that any negative emotions of the week are also flowing out with your breath. Let any feelings of irritation, resentment, fear and anxiety just flow out with your breath, so that you experience a feeling of emptiness before taking the next breath.

The 8:4 Breath

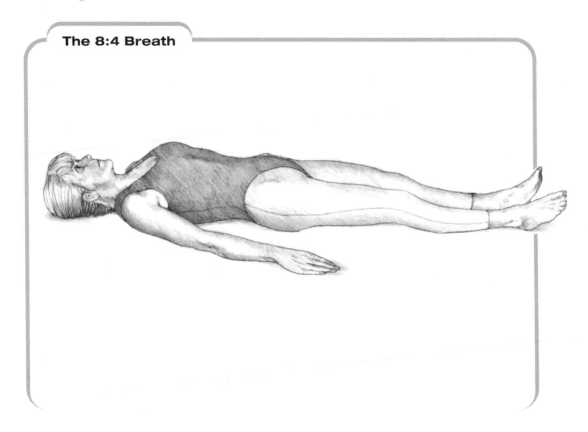

9. The 8:4 Breath

1. Lie on the floor, with your legs flopped apart, and your arms along the side of your body.

2. Watch your breath coming in and out through your nose slowly, and note whether your inhalation is the same length as your exhalation. Pause at the end of each breath, and before the start of your next breath.

3. Inhale slowly for the count of four, and then exhale strongly through your nose, for the count of eight.

4. Really push your breath out through your nose. This may feel strange at first, but visualize your lungs emptying completely with your exhalation, so that it is easier to breathe in the next time.

5. Repeat for seven breaths, inhaling for the count of four, and exhaling for the count of eight.

6. Return to your normal breathing pattern.

Chapter Seven

Routine 5— Parathyroids, Pineal and Pituitary Glands

(Approximately 20 minutes)

This routine builds strength and flexibility in the neck and shoulders to release tension, promote better circulation and prevent stiffness in the joints. This flexibility in the upper body is required to practice postures that put pressure on the pituitary gland in the brain and the parathyroid glands, which lie at the back of the thyroid gland in the throat. The pituitary acts as a feedback system for many of the major glands in the body, and any irregularities in this gland can create a multitude of health problems. The parathyroids are responsible for maintaining the calcium levels in the blood, for strong healthy nerves and bones.

This routine also works on the pineal gland, which produces estrogen-like substances at menopause, to counteract falling levels of estrogen from the ovaries. The Tibetan Lift, Seated Fish and the Elephant are also excellent weight-bearing postures for improving bone strength.

STRETCH

1. Pelvic Floor Lift

Benefits: This lift improves bone strength in the shoulders and ankles, which support the body weight. It strengthens the pelvic floor muscles, to prevent incontinence as we age.

Focus: on using the strength of your thighs to arch your hips higher.

1. Lie on the floor, bend your knees, and clasp your ankles, drawing them in close to your buttocks.

2. Pinch your shoulder blades together, push up onto the top of your shoulders, and arch your hips high to the ceiling. Place your chin on your chest.

3. Squeeze your tummy and buttock muscles tightly.

4. Breathe slowly, while holding the squeeze for a count of seven.

5. Release, by lowering your hips to the floor.

6. While still holding onto your ankles, repeat this squeeze and lower technique seven times.

Pelvic Floor Lift

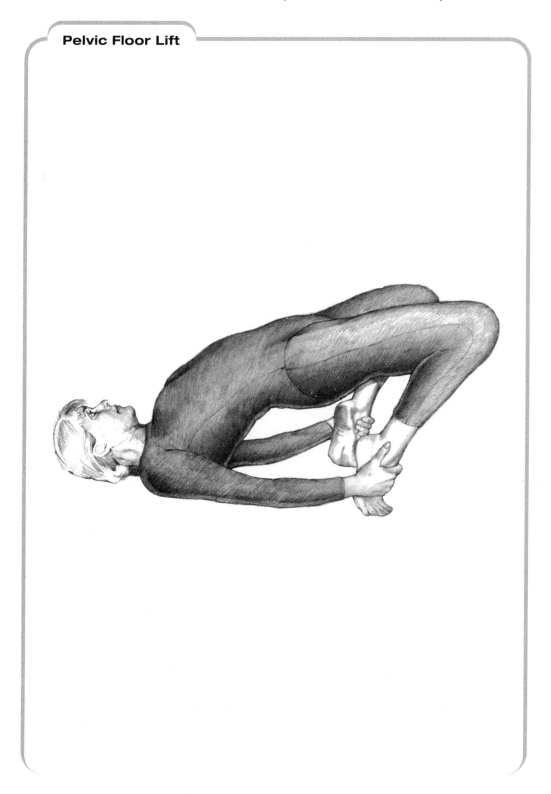

2. Upper Body Lift

Benefits: This lift releases tension in the shoulders and stretches the spine, to open up the vertebrae and improve flexibility.

Focus: on squeezing your shoulder blades tightly together and lifting as much of your upper body off the floor as possible.

1. Lie on your stomach, clasp your hands behind your back, and rest them on your buttocks.

2. Inhale, pinch your shoulder blades together, and lift your upper body off the floor.

3. Lift your arms off your buttocks as high as possible.

4. Breathe slowly, and hold the squeeze for seven counts.

5. Release, and lower to the floor. Repeat seven times.

Upper Body Lift

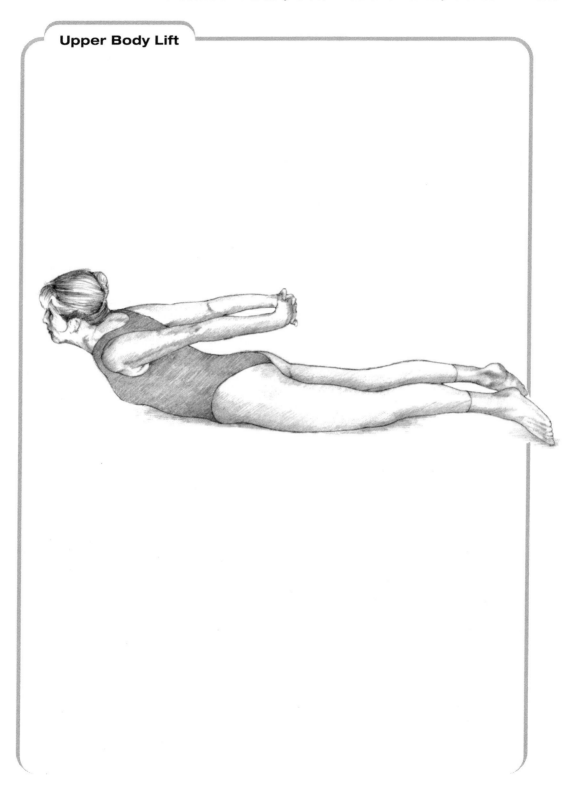

3. Seated Cobra

Benefits: This stretch not only strengthens the shoulder muscles and releases tension, but also creates a lock over the thymus gland in the chest, and restricts the circulation to this area. On releasing the stretch, the gland is flushed with fresh oxygenated blood, to nourish and improve the functioning of the immune system.

Focus: on arching your back strongly, while pushing your hands to the floor and opening up the front of your body.

1. Kneel on the floor with knees apart and your toes tucked under.

2. Clasp your hands behind your back.

3. Inhale, pinch your shoulder blades together, and drop your head right back.

4. Slowly stretch your clasped hands right down to touch the floor, while keeping your balance, and arch through your spine.

5. Breathe slowly, and squeeze your shoulder blades together firmly, while holding the squeeze for the count of seven.

6. Release, by bringing your hands off the floor, and rest your chin on your chest.

7. Repeat.

Seated Cobra

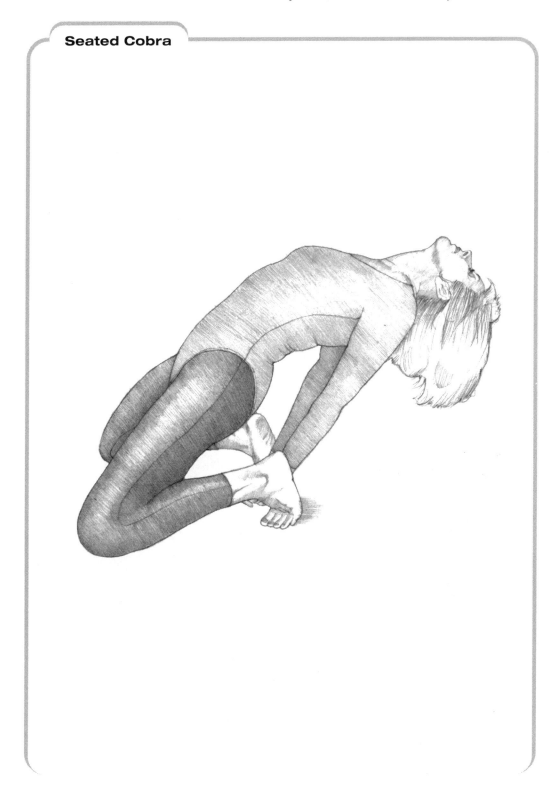

4. Right-Angled Stretch

Benefits: This strong stretch opens up the shoulder joint, improves flexibility of the spine, and improves the strength of the upper arm muscles.

Focus: on getting your chest as close to the floor as possible and keeping your thighs at right angles to the floor.

1. Kneel on the floor, and then sit on your heels, with your arms stretched out in front on the floor. Place your forehead on the floor.

2. Slide your hands away, so that your buttocks lift up off your heels and your thighs are at right angles to the floor.

3. Rest your chin on the floor, and drop your chest close to the floor. Feel the stretch in your upper arms, shoulders, and spine.

4. Arch your back strongly, and breathe slowly seven times in this position. Release, by sliding back onto your heels.

5. Repeat.

ENERGIZE

These postures use the strength and flexibility of the shoulders and upper arms, to support the body and create a lock over the parathyroids. Situated deep within the thyroid gland are several pairs of tiny glands called the parathyroids, which monitor and balance the calcium levels in the blood. These glands are necessary for strong healthy nerves and bones and regular sleep patterns. Too little calcium in the bloodstream results in ragged nerves, erratic moods, and jumpiness that triggers the parathyroids to withdraw calcium from the bones in order to keep the nerves functioning. The Fish and Seated Fish postures work on improving the function of the parathyroids in the side of the neck. This ensures that the right amount of hormones are secreted into the bloodstream, so that excessive calcium is not withdrawn from the bones, resulting in thinning bones.

5. The Fish

This is an excellent posture to use after a frazzled day at the office or in the home, as it immediately calms the nervous system.

Benefits: This posture places a lock over the parathyroids, to promote calcium balance in the body, for strong nerves and bones. It enhances the functioning of the pituitary in the brain, which monitors the functions of many other glands in the body.

Right-Angled Stretch

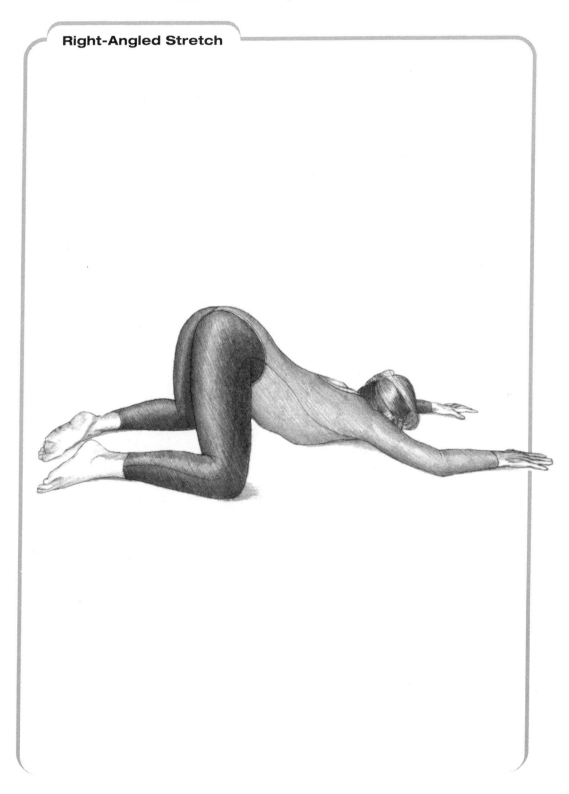

Focus: on pushing on your elbows, to increase the arch in your back and the lock over your throat. Do not try to hold your head up. Let it just hang, to put more pressure on these glands.

Visualize: In both the Fish and the Seated Fish, see yourself as having strong healthy bones and aging well, with good mobility throughout life. Visualize yourself developing an inner calmness and serenity, as you age with strong healthy nerves.

1. Lie on the floor, roll over onto your left hip, and slide your right hand, palms down, under your right buttock.

2. Roll over to your right hip, and slide your left hand, palm down, under your buttock.

3. Cross your thumbs under your buttocks, and sit on your crossed thumbs on the floor.

4. Pinch your shoulder blades together, inhale, and push on your elbows, to lift your head and shoulders off the floor. Your feet will slide away.

5. Let your head hang between your shoulders, to create a lock over the parathyroids in the side of your neck, and restrict the circulation.

6. Breathe slowly for seven breaths.

7. Keep your chest strongly arched, and push on your elbows, to increase the arch in your spine.

8. To release, lower your head to the floor, and flatten the back of your neck.

9. Release your hands from under your body and rest them, palms upward, and relax for a few minutes. Note the feeling of calmness in your body, as this posture works to calm your nervous system.

The Fish

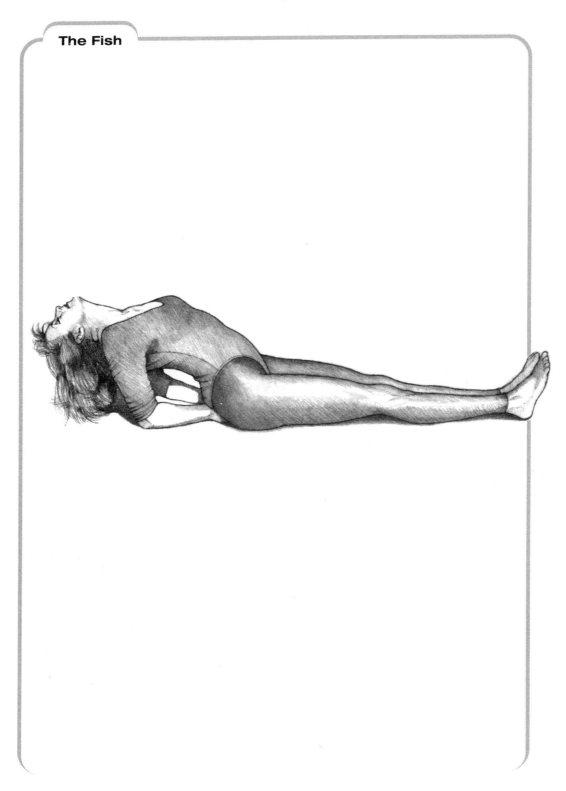

6. Tibetan Lift

Benefits: This strong lift works on the parathyroid gland, to improve calcium balance in the nerves and bones. It also strengthens the pelvic floor muscles, to prevent incontinence in later life.

Focus: on squeezing your shoulder blades together and pushing up from your palms on the floor, to create a higher arch in your spine.

Visualize: See yourself with strong stomach and pelvic floor muscles supporting all of the inner organs, to prevent a prolapse or incontinence as you age.

1. Sit on the floor, with your legs outstretched. Place your hands, palms down, beside your hips.

2. Inhale, bend your knees, lift your hips into the air, and drop your head right back between your shoulders.

3. Squeeze your stomach and buttock muscles tightly, while holding the squeeze for seven counts.

4. To release, exhale through your mouth, lower your hips, straighten your legs, and drop your chin onto your chest.

5. Repeat seven times.

Tibetan Lift

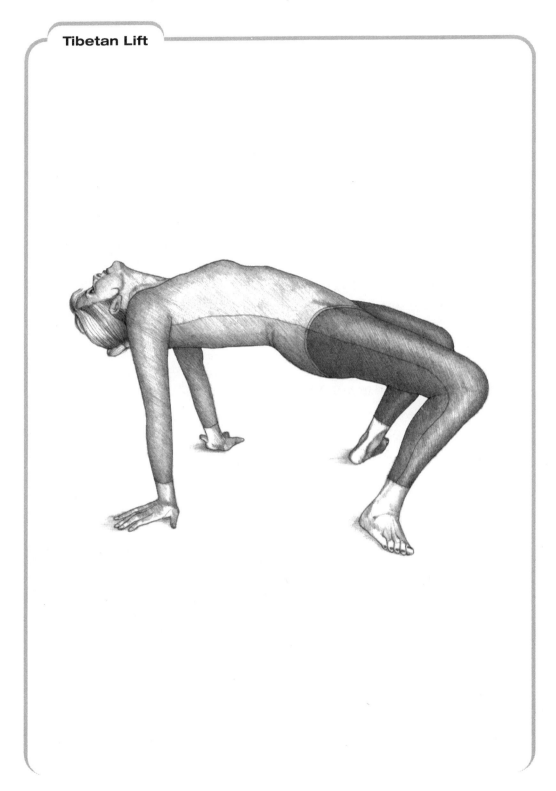

7. Seated Fish

Benefits: This creates a strong lock over the parathyroids, to improve calcium balance, as well as strengthening the bones of the arms and legs.

Focus: on pushing your toes into the floor, while lifting your hips higher.

1. Sit on the floor, with your legs stretched out in front, and your palms flat on the floor beside you.

2. Adjust your fingers, so that they are pointing away from your body.

3. Take your weight onto your hands, and lift your hips upward.

4. Balance on your arms and hands, with your elbows locked.

5. Pinch your shoulder blades together, drop your head back, and point your toes to the floor for support.

6. Breathe slowly in and out through your nose, as you hold this position for three breaths.

7. To return, lower your hips to the seated position, and take a deep slow breath.

8. Repeat this position two more times, as you visualize your wrist, forearm and upper arms becoming stronger.

9. To release, lie back on the floor and breathe slowly.

Seated Fish

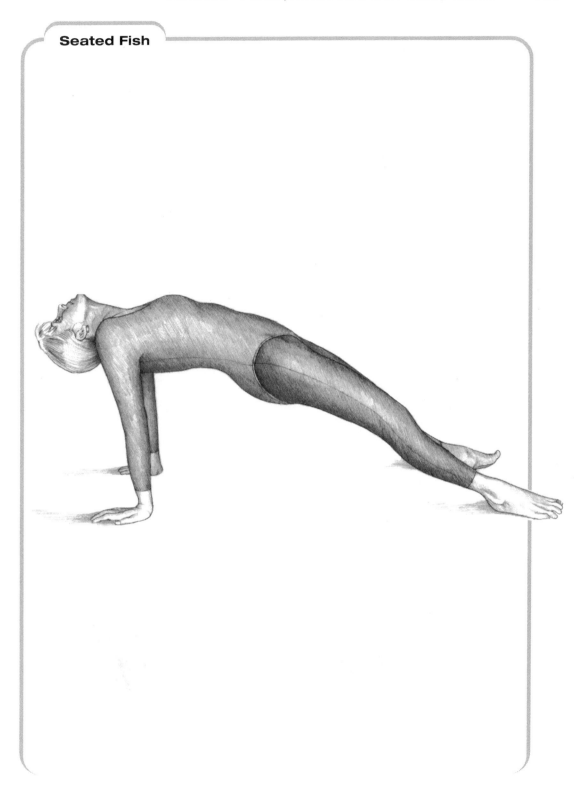

8. The Elephant

This posture puts pressure on the pineal gland located centrally and high in the brain. This gland produces estrogen-like substances at menopause, to balance the body's falling estrogen levels from the ovaries. Postures that work on this gland in yoga include those that place pressure on the head by inverting the body, such as the Elephant, as described below, and the Crane postures.

Recent studies have revealed that this very light-sensitive gland is crucial in the balancing of depression and manic states, and in the prevention of "winter blues." The pineal is the master gland that is responsible for our body rhythms and our moods. When it is stable, this gland will allow all of the other glands to be in balance in the body and function as they should.

Benefits: In this position, the heart does not have to pump against gravity for the blood to reach the brain, so the heart is rested. The spine is stretched, as well as the hamstrings. Pressure is placed on the pineal gland, for better functioning of all of the glandular system, especially the glands concerned with moods.

Focus: on lengthening and stretching through your spine, so that your head comes lower to the floor.

Visualize: See yourself moving serenely through life, with balanced moods and the right balance of hormones needed by your body.

1. Kneel on all fours on the floor, with your hands shoulder-width apart, and your feet hip-width apart. Tuck your toes under.

2. Move your body weight forward into your hands, and push your hips up to the ceiling, while straightening your legs.

3. Stretch through your spine, with your head hanging loosely between your shoulders.

4. Move your weight into the back of your heels, by pushing on the palms of your hands, and breathe slowly seven times.

5. To release, move your weight forward onto your hands again, step your feet together, and bend your knees.

6. Sit back on your heels and rest, before coming into a seated position.

Elephant

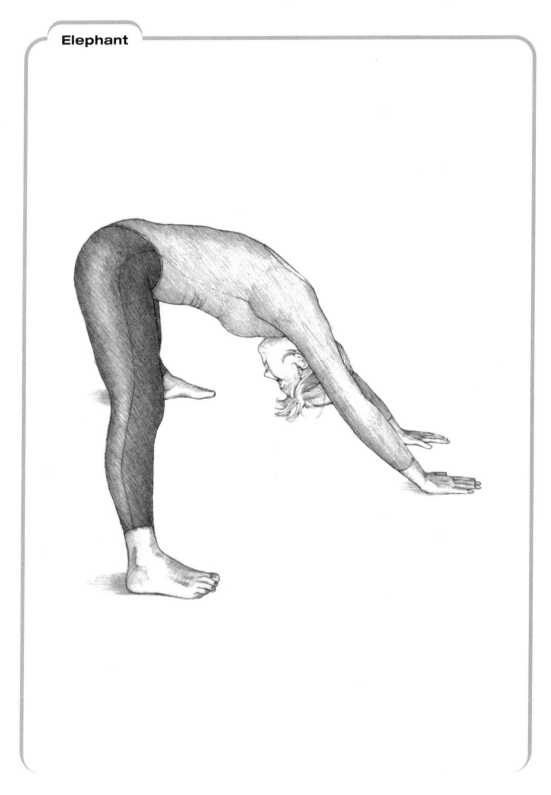

BREATHE

9. The Ha Breath

Benefits: This strong breathing technique releases tension in the neck and shoulders, while getting rid of excess carbon dioxide in the body, which can cause fatigue.

Focus: on forcefully breathing out, and making the "ha" sound strongly. Stretch your arms as far away as possible on the forward stretch.

1. Lie on the floor, with your arms stretched above your head, shoulder-width apart, and your legs wide.

2. Inhale through your nose, then exhale forcefully through your mouth, saying "ha," while bending your knees and coming into a sitting position, with your feet on the floor.

3. Push your outstretched arms through your knees, and stretch through your spine.

4. Inhale, stretch your arms overhead, and lie down again, while straightening your legs. Your arms should be shoulder-width apart on the floor, above your head.

5. Repeat seven times.

The Ha Breath

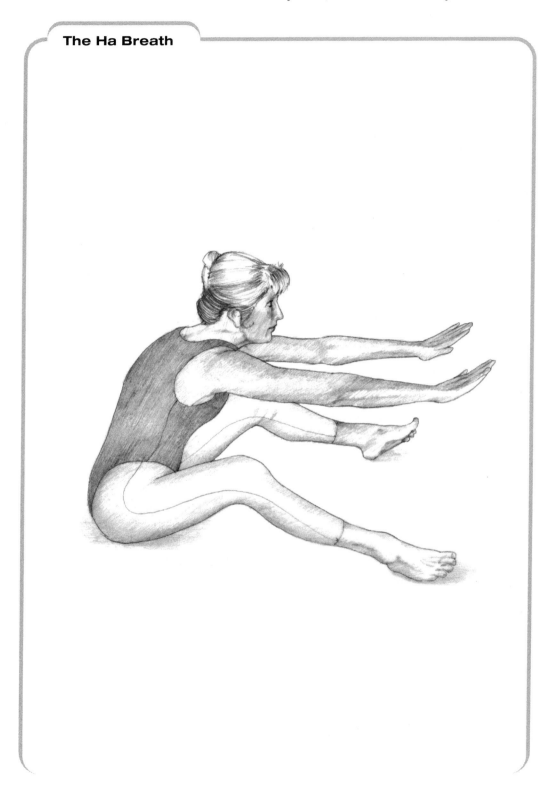

Summary

The five routines from Chapters 3–7 have been designed to build both muscle and bone strength evenly throughout the upper and lower body. For best results you need to practice a selection of stretches, postures and breathing techniques from each of the routines. The combination of techniques is unlimited and will depend on your needs and time limitations.

To begin: Assess your upper body strength using the exercises in Chapter 1: Beyond Calcium.

Practice the Full Yoga Breath in Chapter 2: Getting Started.

Select and practice 2-3 warm up stretches from Chapter 2: Getting Started.

Select and practice one stretch and one energizing posture from each of the routines below:

> Chapter 3: Routine 1—Upper Body
> Chapter 4: Routine 2—Lower Body
> Chapter 5: Routine 3—The Ovaries
> Chapter 6: Routine 4—The Adrenals
> Chapter 7: Routine 5—The Parathyroids
> Focus on the visualization given for each stretch or posture.

Ideally set aside 20 minutes each day to work on building muscle and bone strength to prevent the onset of osteoporosis. For example, a typical workout to build muscle and bone strength may include the following:

> Chapter 2: Getting Started—Tabletop, Squats and Spine Curl
> Chapter 3: Upper Body—Stretch: Wall Rotation, Energizing Posture:
> The Wedge
> Chapter 4: Lower Body—Stretch: Squats, Energizing Posture:
> Balancing Spine Twist
> Chapter 5: Ovaries—Stretch: Spine Twist, Energizing Posture: Bent Leg
> Creative Power Posture
> Chapter 6: The Adrenals—Stretch: Hip Rolls, Energizing Posture:
> Bow In Cat Posture
> Chapter 7: The Parathyroids—Stretch: Pelvic Floor Lift, Energizing
> Posture: The Fish
> To finish: Chapter 2: Getting Started
> 7 rounds of Full Yoga Breath

Note: Use a similar approach when selecting the techniques for menopausal relief.

Chapter *Eight*

Special Yoga Techniques for Menopausal Symptom Relief

On average, two-thirds of women go through menopause with very little disruption to their lives. One-third suffer no symptoms, one-third suffer mild or occasional symptoms, and the other third suffer severe symptoms, which can disrupt their family and work lives. The following techniques address five of the most common complaints throughout menopause, which yoga can help alleviate: mood swings, lack of energy, lack of concentration and mental fuzziness, weight gain, and disrupted sleep patterns.

MOOD SWINGS

A number of yoga postures balance the reproductive glands, by creating a lock over the ovaries that are responsible for our monthly cycles, sexuality, creativity, and aging. Having more regular cycles means having more even levels of estrogen and progesterone, for maintaining strong healthy bones. It also means more balanced moods and improved creative energy, which can be used for pursuits that interest us. When we are creatively employed, we often lose ourselves in our activity, which heightens our moods. Libido is improved with regular cycles and balanced levels of reproductive hormones, and sexual activity is one of nature's greatest mood enhancers. It releases "feel good" chemicals, called endorphins, to the brain. Yoga postures keep the reproductive glands, which produce and reproduce every cell in our body, nourished and free of toxins, so that we do not age prematurely. All of these benefits will certainly enhance our moods.

1. Half-Lotus Creative Power Posture

This simple forward-bending creative power posture creates a lock over the reproductive glands, and restricts the circulation to this area. By breathing deeply in the position, the ovaries are supplied with extra oxygen to nourish and repair all the cells of the body. As the position is released, the body is flushed with fresh oxygenated blood to nourish and energize these glands.

Benefits: This posture stretches right throughout the spine, as well as through the back of the hamstrings of the outstretched leg. It puts pressure on the large artery in the top of the thigh, so that more blood flow is directed upward to the brain, for clear thinking. It refreshes and nourishes the reproductive organs for healthy functioning.

Focus: on creating a strong squeeze over your groin, by bringing your chest closer to your thighs.

1. Sit on the floor, with your legs outsretched.
2. Bend your right knee and take hold of your foot, guiding it as high as possible onto the top of your left thigh, with the sole of your foot turned upward.
3. Flex the toes of your left foot toward your body, and place your hands, palms down, beside your hips.
4. Inhale, stretch both arms above your head, and lift up through your rib cage, stretching through both sides of your spine.
5. Keeping the length in your spine, exhale, bend forward, and clasp your left ankle firmly, with your elbows bent and your forearms as close to the floor as possible.
6. While holding onto your ankle, inhale, and stretch your spine upward, while straightening your elbows.
7. Exhale, bend your elbows, and draw your upper body down close to your thighs, squeezing into your groin area.
8. Repeat this stretch-and-squeeze movement for three breaths.

Half-Lotus Creative Power Posture

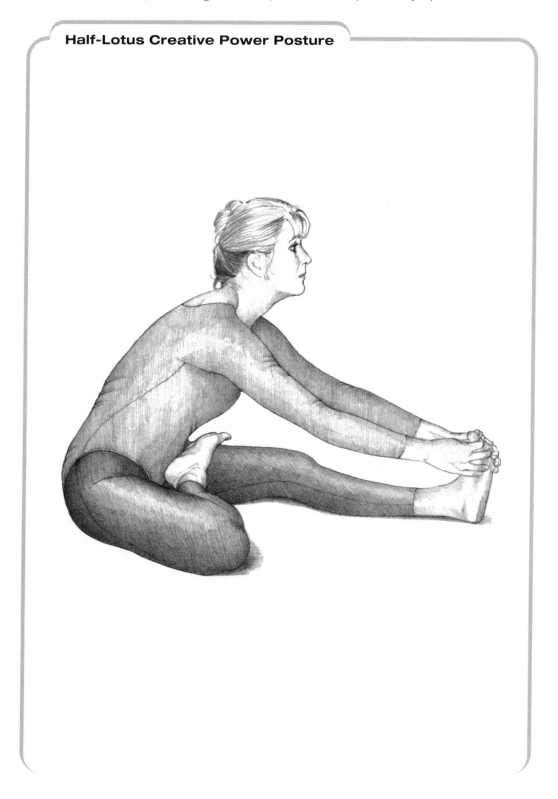

9. To release, stretch your hands forward and up above your head, and release them in a wide circle, back to the side of your body.

10. Change sides, and repeat three times on the other side.

On completion of the posture, bend your knees and clasp your hands around your knees. Rock your body backward and forward onto your back, to release any strain in your lower back.

2. The Tree

This balancing posture takes time to master. You can practice it more easily, first thing in the morning, when your mind is quiet, before the emotional ups and downs of the day disturb your peace of mind.

Benefits: This balancing posture builds strength in the bones of each leg, as it bears the entire body weight on one leg. It also improves concentration and induces a calm mental state.

Focus: on a point in front of you, and on keeping your supporting leg locked at the knee, to stop any wobbling. Lift up through your rib cage, to lengthen your spine and help keep your balance. Use the wall for balance, if necessary.

1. Stand sideways, about an arm-width away from a wall, with your left hip parallel to the wall. Place your legs hip-width apart.

2. Move your weight onto your left foot, and slide your right foot up high into the inside of your left inner thigh. Use your hands to position your foot firmly in place.

3. Pull up through your left kneecap, to lock your leg firmly.

4. Place your hands in prayer-position, palms together in front of your chest, and steady your balance.

5. Breathe evenly, and gaze at a spot on the floor, to hold your concentration steady.

6. Once balanced, take your arms in a wide arc above your head, and clasp your hands together, with the first finger of each hand joined and pointing upward, like a steeple.

7. Keep your left leg locked, and pull your right knee back a little, so that your body is in a flat plane. Lift up through your rib cage, to stay steady.

8. Hold your balance, and, focusing on a point in front of you, breathe seven times. To release, lower your right leg to the floor.

9. Turn your right hip to the wall, and repeat on your other side, holding the position for seven breaths.

The Tree

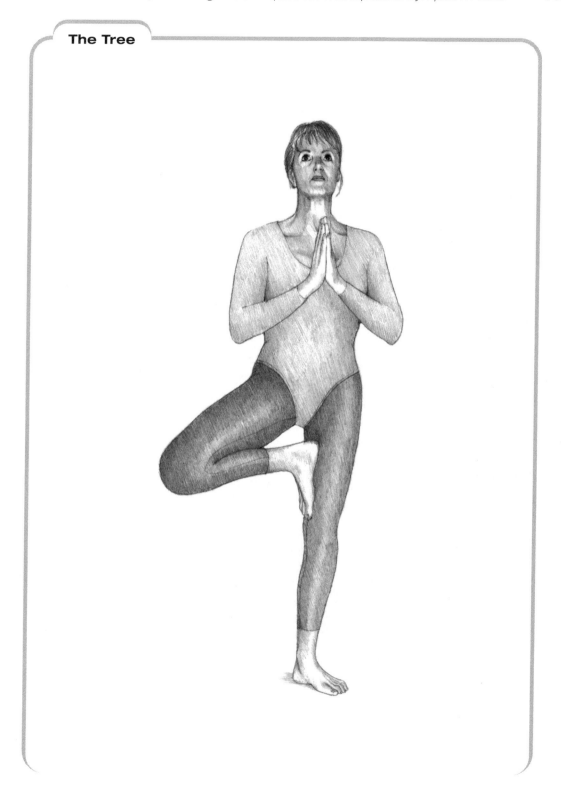

3. The Crane

Note: This posture is not recommended for those with neck or shoulder problems, unless under the guidance of an experienced yoga teacher.

Benefits: This posture puts pressure on the pituitary gland in the brain, the master gland, which acts as a feedback system in the human body. It monitors the activities of the lower glands, and triggers adjustments via the hormones it produces, to keep the system stable. It is often referred to as the most complex chemical factory in the body, because of its myriad secretions and the effects they trigger. These glands are responsible for keeping moods, appetites and sleep patterns in balance.

Focus: on smooth, steady, step-by-step movements, which do not upset your balance. Do not progress to the next step until you feel comfortable. The closer your head is to your toes in this position, the easier it is to balance, so do not step your feet away from your head when you straighten your legs.

1. Kneel on the floor, and bring your elbows around the outside of your knees. Interlace your fingers, making a triangle on the floor.

2. Place the crown of your head inside the triangle, resting on the flat spot on your head.

3. Tuck your toes under, and release your hands to the outside of your knees (about 10" away), with your elbows bent and your palms flat on the floor.

4. Keeping your head, hands, and feet in this position, push your hips to the ceiling and straighten your legs. Do not step your feet away.

5. Step your legs wide apart, until each leg is near an elbow.

6. Bend your right knee, and rest it on your elbow. Slowly bend your other knee, and place it on your elbow, bringing the soles of your feet together, to complete the balance.

7. Straighten up through your neck, by pulling your shoulders away from your ears.

8. Breathe slowly in the position for three breaths.

9. To release, step one foot down to the floor, then the other, and step your feet together.

10. Bend your knees and sit on your heels, while resting your head on your clenched fists. Take a couple of breaths, and then return to the seated position.

The Crane

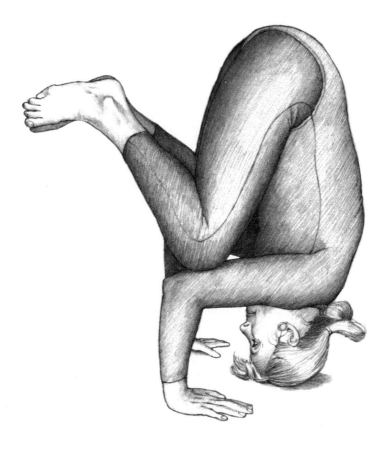

4. A 10-Minute Yoga Mini-Workout: Salute to the Sun

Symbolically, this sequence works to draw in energy from the sun, so that it can be used for the highest purposes throughout the day. Ideally, this posture should be done outside, first thing in the morning. Since this is not always convenient, particularly in certain climates, you can work indoors, and visualize recharging your body with each step.

Benefits: Salute to the Sun is an ancient yoga workout that is designed to stretch and tone all of the muscles and joints, strengthen the bones, improve breathing and heart rate, improve concentration, cleanse the glandular system of toxins, and lift depression and anxiety. Because of the way it creates a lock over various glands to balance hormone levels, it increases energy levels, calms moods, and balances the metabolic rate for weight maintenance. It consists of 12 steps, and can be practiced as fast as you like, either in an aerobic workout, or more slowly and gracefully. Make sure that you warm up first, with the stretches in the earlier "Getting Started" section.

Focus: on keeping your movements smooth and graceful, and your breathing even and rhythmic.

Visualize: See yourself able to cope with the ups and downs of each day and still remain cheerful, so that you don't waste emotional energy by needlessly reacting or overreacting to others around you. See yourself being inwardly calm and serene, while you breathe deeply throughout each of the steps in the sequence.

Step 1

1. Stand with your feet hip-width apart, and your palms together in front of your chest.
2. Inhale, and take your arms in a wide circle out to the side, and join your palms overhead.
3. Exhale, and return your palms to your chest. Release your hands to the side of your body.

Step 2

Inhale, extend your arms overhead, and arch back. This creates a lock over the parathyroids, for calcium balance. It also creates a lock over the adrenals, which control stress levels and take over the production of estrogen-like substances at menopause.

Step 3

Exhale, bend forward, and place both of your palms on either side of your feet. Tuck your chin under. This creates a lock over the thyroid gland, for balancing the metabolic rate. It also creates a lock over the ovaries, for balancing estrogen and progesterone levels.

Salute to the Sun—Steps 1, 2, and 3

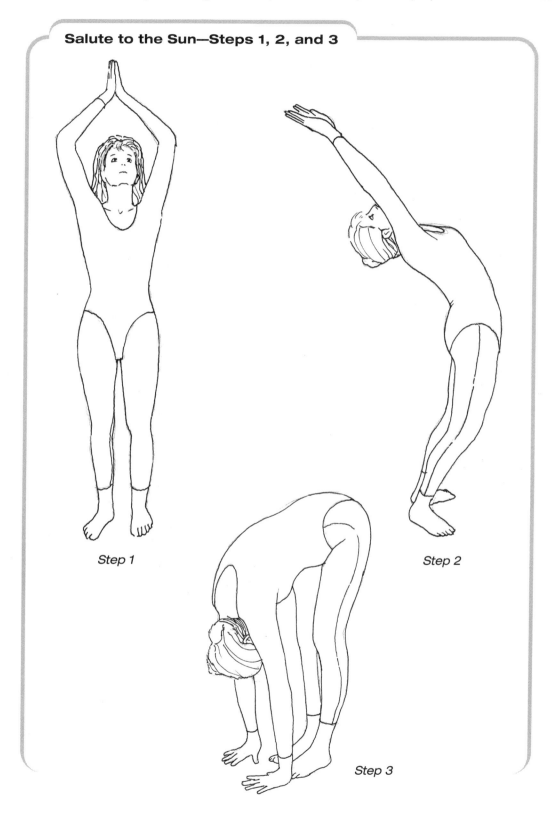

Step 1

Step 2

Step 3

Step 4

1. Inhale, and step your left leg back, bringing your left knee to the floor.

2. Bend your right knee in a forward lunge. Extend through your chin. This massages the internal organs, to encourage elimination.

Step 5

1. Exhale, and extend your right leg back.

2. Tighten your stomach muscles, while supporting your body weight on your locked arms and toes.

Step 6

1. Hold your breath, drop to your knees, and sit back on your heels.

2. Place your hands, chin, and chest on the floor, with a strong arch in your lower back. This creates a lock over the suprarenal glands that control stress levels.

Salute to the Sun—Steps 4, 5, and 6

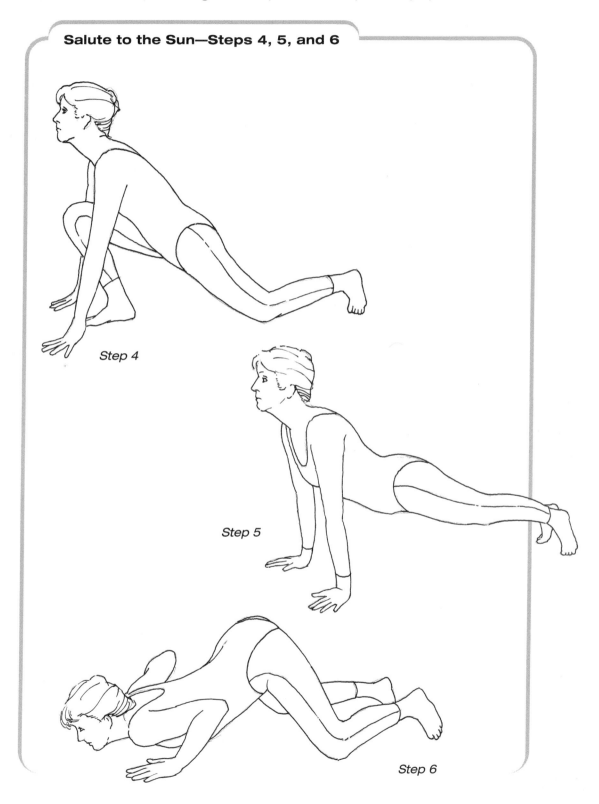

Step 4

Step 5

Step 6

Step 7

1. Inhale, lift your elbows, and slide your body forward through your hands and upward.

2. Drop your pelvis to the floor, and arch back with your legs wide and toes tucked under. This creates a lock over the thymus gland, to balance the immune system.

Step 8

1. Exhale, push up onto your feet and hands, and drop your head through your shoulders.

2. Push your hips into the air, forming an inverted "V" position, and stretch your heels to the floor. This puts pressure on the pituitary and pineal glands in the brain, which controls appetites, sleep, patterns, moods, sexuality, and intelligence. It also increases blood supply to the head, for clear thinking.

Step 9

1. Inhale, and step your left leg forward between your hands.

2. Bend your left leg into a lunge, and bring your right knee to the floor.

3. Look forward, and lengthen along your chest.

Salute to the Sun—Steps 7, 8, and 9

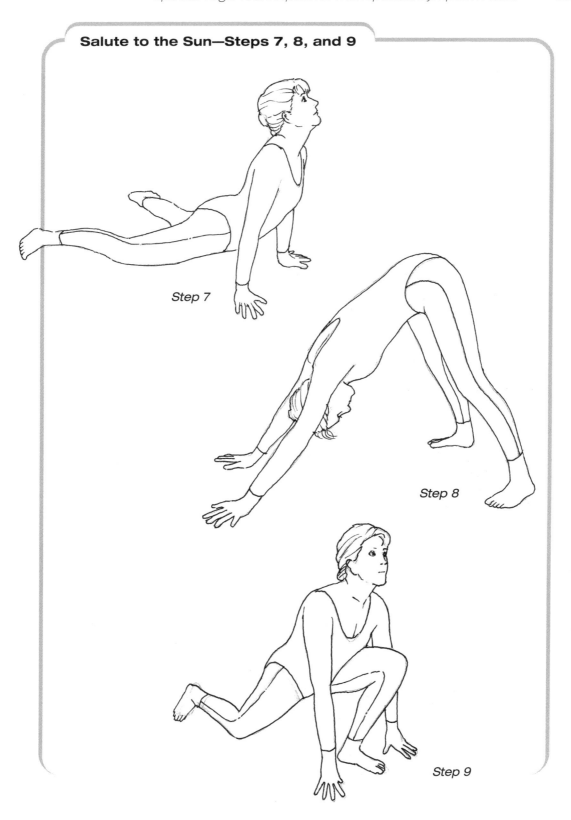

Step 7

Step 8

Step 9

Step 10

1. Exhale, and step your right foot between your hands.

2. Draw your upper body down along your thighs, with your chin tucked under.

3. Straighten both legs, creating a lock in the thyroid gland in the throat to control your body's metabolic rate.

Step 11

1. Inhale, stretch your arms forwards, raise them overhead, and arch backwards with your head back.

2. Exhale, and take your arms in a wide circle, down along the outside of your thighs. Drop your head back, with your back arched strongly.

Step 12

1. Inhale, and bring your hands in a wide circle again, above your head.

2. Exhale, and return your hands to prayer-position in front of your chest.

3. Close your eyes, take a deep, slow breath, and release your hands to the side of your body.

4. Repeat six more sequences of these 12 steps.

On Completion of the Salute to the Sun

1. Stand quietly, while your heart rate and breath come back to normal.

2. Lock your knees, and pull your stomach muscles in.

3. Tuck your buttock muscles under, and lift up through your rib cage, while lengthening in your spine.

4. Lift your shoulders up, back, and down, and bring your chin level with the floor.

5. Feel as if someone is pulling you up from a string in the crown of your head, and lengthen throughout your entire spine, so that your vertebrae align themselves evenly. You are now standing in "perfect posture."

6. Hold this relaxed position for seven slow breaths, open your eyes, and release the position.

Salute to the Sun—Steps 10, 11, and 12

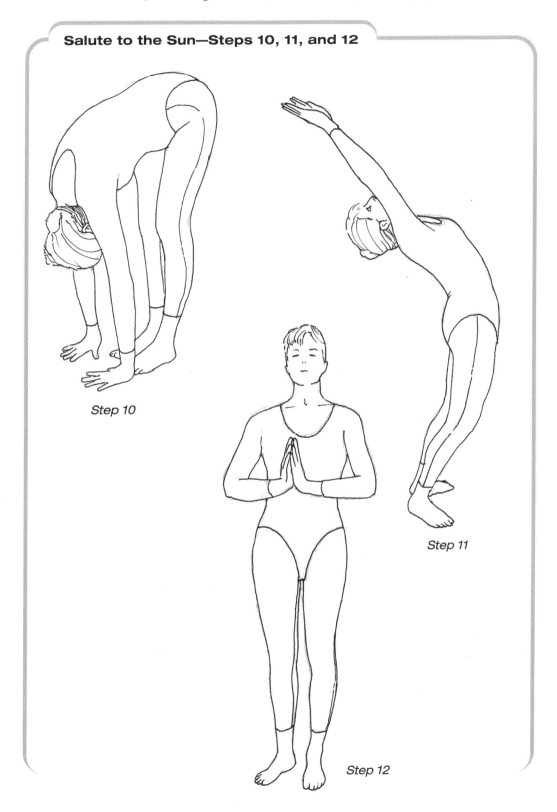

Step 10

Step 11

Step 12

LACK OF ENERGY

A lack of energy is often mistakenly blamed on menopause alone because of slight changes in hormone levels, which can alter moods and the way we feel about life in general. Menopause may not be the only culprit. For example, consider the following causes:

◆ Air-conditioned cars, offices and homes can limit the supply of oxygen to the blood, which slows down the metabolic rate and energy levels. Just as a candle needs oxygen to burn brightly, so we need plenty of oxygen to stay energetic.

◆ Pollution in the air, food, and water supplies overloads our bodies with toxins and makes the liver work harder and become sluggish. Installing a water purifier and eating more organic food can help to offset this condition.

◆ Being overweight causes the heart to work harder and makes us tire more easily. Eating too many fats and sugars also overloads the liver, making it sluggish. The book by Dr. Sandra Cabot, *The Liver Cleansing Diet*, shows how to detoxify the liver and boost energy levels.

◆ Lack of regular exercise limits oxygen supplies to the brain and bloodstream, slowing us down.

◆ Tension in the neck, shoulders, and back muscles from incorrect breathing habits can drain us of energy. Increased tension from continually having to meet deadlines or a perceived lack of time to complete them can leave us feeling tired and lethargic.

◆ The health of the thyroid gland affects energy levels, because it governs the oxygen levels in the blood. If this gland is underactive, the metabolic rate slows down, giving us a feeling of dragging ourselves through the day. If your energy levels are consistently low, coupled with extreme mood swings, have a thyroid blood test.

The following yoga techniques address a lack of energy in the body, which can be caused by a combination of hormonal, lifestyle and environmental factors, but not necessarily a medical cause.

5. Bandha

Benefits: This posture works to improve the functioning of the pancreas, which produces insulin, to balance the sugar levels in the body and thus, energy levels. When the flow of insulin to the body is regulated, the body maintains steady energy levels throughout the day.

Focus: on pulling your stomach muscles up tightly, creating pressure over your pancreas.

1. Stand with your legs wide apart. Bend your knees and squat, with your hands resting on your knees, and your fingertips facing inward.

Bandha

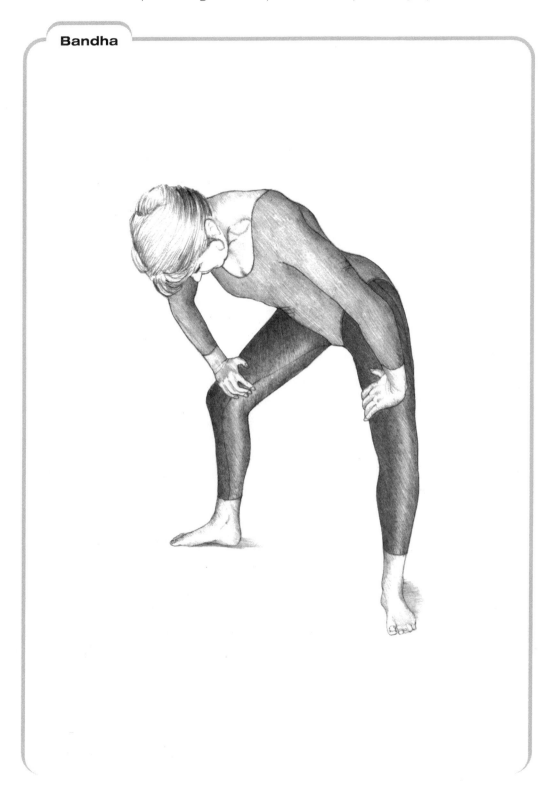

2. Inhale, and exhale forcefully through your open mouth.

3. Close your mouth, tuck your chin into your chest, and hold your breath.

4. Suck your stomach muscles back, up and under your rib cage, and hold your breath for the count of seven.

5. To release, exhale, and straighten your legs. Bend forward, and hang loosely.

6. Repeat twice more.

6. Assisted Shoulder Stand

Note: Do not attempt this posture if you have neck problems, unless you are under the guidance of an experienced yoga teacher.

Benefits: Balancing the entire body weight on the shoulders and upper arms in the shoulder stand creates a lock over the thyroid gland, which regulates oxygen levels in the blood and thus, energy levels. The inverted position also rests the legs and prevents pooling of blood in the large veins, helping to prevent varicose veins and the more serious condition, thrombosis. It also improves balance and clarity of thought by increasing the circulation to the brain, without the heart having to pump against gravity.

Focus: on being as high onto your shoulder blades as possible, in order to take the pressure off your neck. Do not move your head or neck once you are in the position.

Visualize: See yourself with more than enough energy to take you through each day.

1. Lie on your back, with your legs up the wall and your buttocks touching the wall.

2. Bend your knees, and place your feet hip-width apart on the wall. Your hands should be beside your hips, with your palms flat.

3. Inhale, and push your feet against the wall. Arch your back and balance evenly on both shoulder blades.

4. Place your hands behind your waist, with your fingertips pointing toward your spine.

5. Wiggle from side to side, to bring your body weight high onto your shoulders.

6. Move your elbows close together behind your back for support, and breathe slowly to steady your body.

Assisted Shoulder Stand

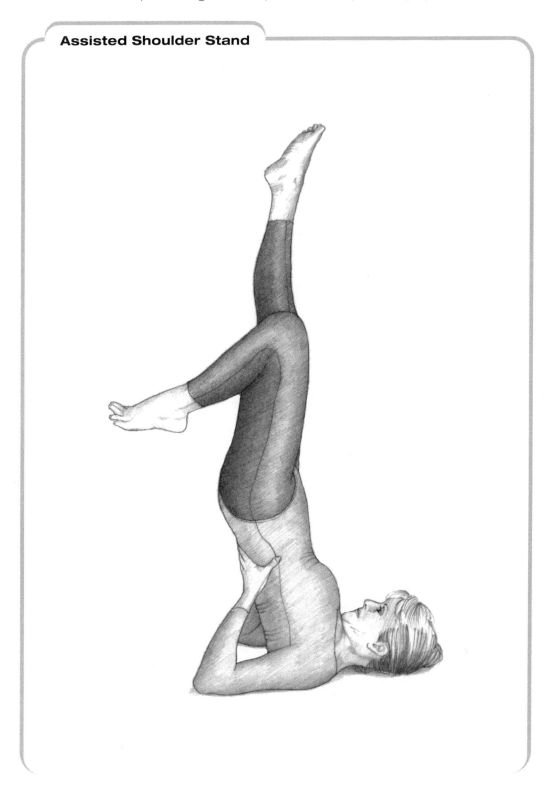

7. Keeping your spine strong and arched, lift one foot of the wall and straighten your leg.

8. Take your weight onto your shoulders, slowly lift your other leg off the wall, and straighten. Do not move your head or neck in this position.

9. Your chin should be firmly on your chest, creating the lock over your throat, to restrict circulation to your thyroid gland.

10. Breathe slowly seven times.

11. To release, lower one foot to the wall, then the other foot, slide your elbows out, and lower your hips to the floor.

12. Rest your legs up the wall. The thyroid gland is now flushed with fresh, oxygenated blood, nourishing it, so that your metabolic rate is not too fast or too slow. Practice this shoulder stand two to three times a week, whenever your energy levels sag.

7. Tapping Breath

This breath needs to be done vigorously, so do not be afraid to tap the bony parts of your chest firmly for best effect. It works to remove toxins in your lungs caused by pollution, and removes congestion caused by infections.

Benefits: This breath is designed to help detoxify the lungs. It has a very stimulating effect on energy levels, as the lungs become cleaner. It is especially good for people who have had a chest infection or for people who are smokers.

Focus: on tapping all over the bony parts of your ribs, but not on the soft breast tissues.

1. Stand with your arms outstretched to shoulder-height and your legs wide apart.

2. Inhale, hold your breath, and drop your head back.

3. With your palms open, start to slap quite firmly in a circle, starting from the side of your ribcage, up onto the bony part of your upper chest, then under your collarbone, down the other side of your ribs, and to the base of your ribs.

4. Exhale, while stretching your arms out to your side at shoulder-height. Then bend forward, letting your body just hang loosely.

5. Without taking a breath in between, inhale again, take the arms to shoulder height and repeat for six more rounds.

6. To release this technique, just bend forward, and hang loosely like a rag doll. Sense how clean and stimulated your lungs feel.

Tapping Breath

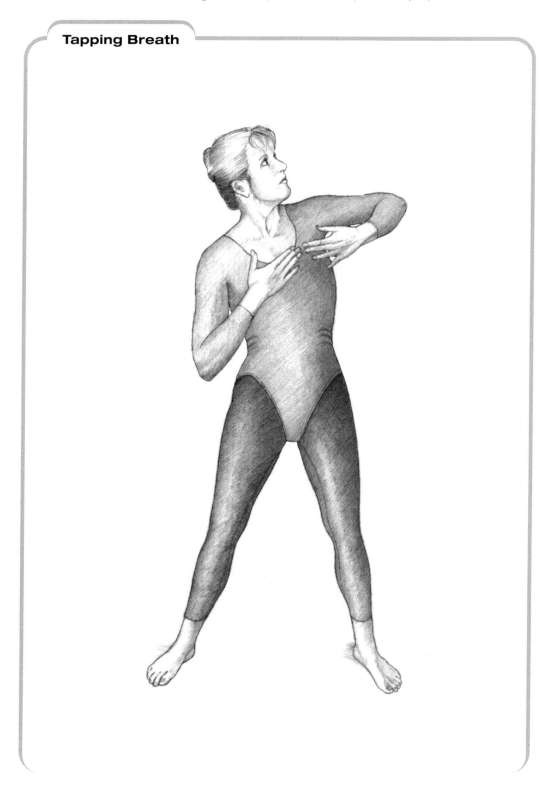

MENTAL FUZZINESS/LACK OF CONCENTRATION

While many women complain of poor memory throughout menopause, this does not necessarily mean that they are candidates for Alzheimer's disease. Our minds function just like a computer, storing and retrieving information, mostly without ever having to think about it. However, in today's highly technological world, we have much to remember, such as pin numbers for banking and shopping, security codes for the office, passwords for computers, mobile phone numbers, e-mail addresses, and many other important numbers. Just as we need to clear out disks in a computer to make space, we sometimes need to offload clutter from the mind, in order to recharge our thinking capacity. If you can't remember where you put the teapot and later find it in the refrigerator, or if you forget where you parked your car at the supermarket, it's time to practice these postures and techniques.

Use the mental clarity and periods of inner stillness that come with the following techniques to consciously reflect on the mental clutter in your life, in your relationships, at work, and at home. Perhaps you are holding onto responsibilities that are no longer yours, or over-committing yourself to things that are not really important to you any longer. You might be spending time going mentally over and over past hurts, using your best energy on things you cannot change. In the quietness that follows the Mudra and breathing technique, ask yourself how you can unclutter your life a little. And then listen, in the silence, for the answer.

8. Mudra

Mudras are ancient sequences traditionally handed down from teacher to student by word of mouth. The combination of equal movement on both sides of the body, deep breathing, and a focus for the mind brings both hemispheres of the brain into balance and harmony.

Benefits: Mudras activate both hemispheres of the brain: the left, or logical side, and the right, or creative side, so that you can operate effectively on both sides.

Focus: on making smooth and graceful movements and a feeling of humbleness in this position. Keep breathing when your head is bowed toward the floor.

Note: If you find difficulty in taking your head to the floor, use a rolled towel under your buttocks, so that your head can touch the floor.

1. Sit in a comfortable cross-legged position on the floor

2. Pull out your buttock muscles from underneath you so that you are sitting firmly on the floor, with your hips tilted forward a little, and your spine gently arched.

Mudra

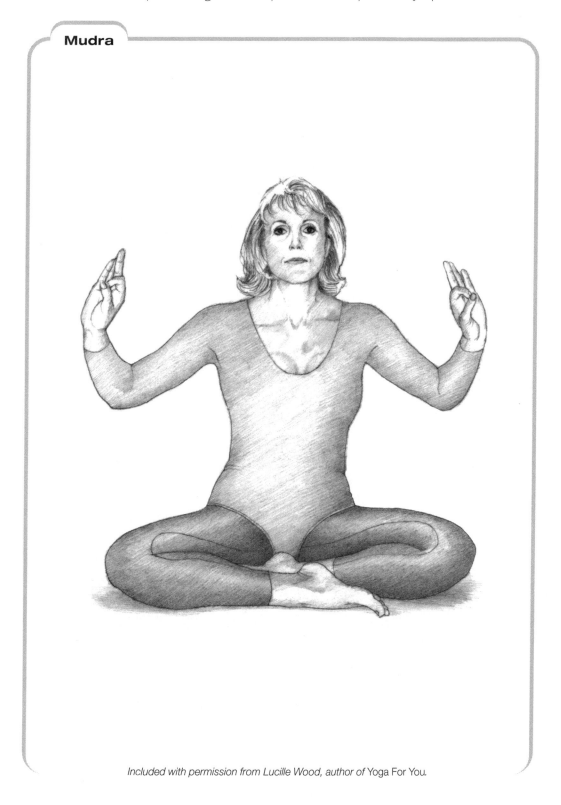

Included with permission from Lucille Wood, author of Yoga For You.

3. Curl your thumb and first finger together in the OM position, and place the backs of the hands on the knees.

4. Inhale, take both arms out to the side at shoulder height and bend your elbows.

5. Exhale, bend forward taking the arms behind the back, crossing the wrists. Rest the wrists on the back.

6. Drop your head as close to the floor as possible and pause.

7. Inhale, and return the arms to the side at shoulder height.

8. Exhale, and return the backs of the hands to the knees and pause.

9. Repeat three times.

The mudra is always done three times. For the first time, focus on respect for yourself; all that you are, can be and will be in this lifetime. For the second time, focus on respect for others; for all that they are, can be and will be in this lifetime. For the third time, focus on respect for the universal energy that we all share.

9. Standing Spine Twist

Benefits: This releases trapped muscles and nerves, so that the messages from the central nervous system can flow freely between the brain and the body without obstruction, so you are more alert and focused.

Focus: on the openness of your shoulders and spine, and on rotating your body into one flat plane.

Visualize: See yourself with a flexible spine, able to move in any direction. Also see yourself as being neither too accommodating, nor too rigid. See yourself able to react quickly and positively to life's opportunities.

1. Stand with your feet wide apart and your arms stretched out to shoulder-height. Look to the right, and turn your right foot out and your left foot slightly inward.

2. Inhale, then exhale, and lean over to the right, stretching your arm parallel to the floor.

3. Drop your right hand to your right ankle, and clasp it firmly.

4. Turn, twist, and look up as you inhale, and extend your left arm up to the ceiling at right angles to your body.

5. Exhale, and pull your left hip and shoulder back, to rotate your spine and make space between your vertebrae for energy to flow freely up and down your spine. Breathe steadily three times.

Standing Spine Twist

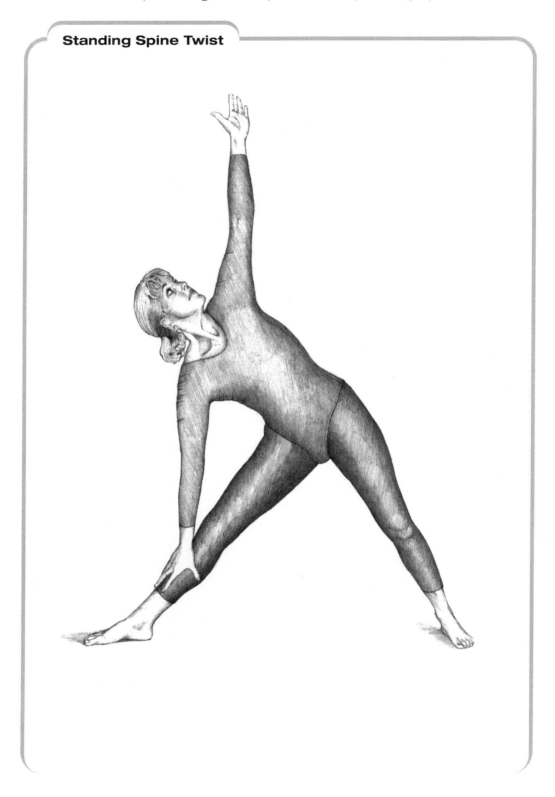

6. To return, look down at your right hand, inhale, and come back to the starting position.

7. Turn your right foot in, your left foot out, and repeat on the other side, holding the position for three breaths.

10. Alternate Nostril Breath

This is a wonderful breath for clearing your mind of thoughts that flutter, like a butterfly, from one topic to another all day long. The extra oxygen it brings to your brain clears your focus and brings clarity back into your mind. It is particularly good for restoring emotional calm after an argument!

Benefits: This technique works to bring equal amounts of oxygen to both sides of the brain, for effective mental functioning in both the logical and creative aspects of the mind. It improves focus and concentration, calms the nerves, and creates mental stillness.

Focus: on making your inhalations and exhalations the same length. Feel as if your whole body is centered over your coccyx bone at the base of your spine, and feel your emotions calm down and your mind clear, as you practice this breath

1. Sit in a comfortable, cross-legged position, with your hands resting on your knees. Your spine should be upright, but relaxed.

2. Place the first two fingers of your right hand firmly on the crook of your nose.

3. Rest your right thumb on your right nostril, and your ring finger on your left nostril.

4. Close your right nostril with your thumb, and inhale slowly through your left nostril.

5. Close your left nostril with your ring finger, and exhale through your right nostril.

6. Breathe back in through your right nostril, close it, and breathe out through your left nostril. This completes one round.

7. Repeat for six more rounds.

Remember that if you find yourself breathing in, you should close that nostril and breathe out through your other nostril. If you find yourself breathing out, breathe back in through that same nostril, close it, and breathe out through the other one.

Alternate Nostril Breath

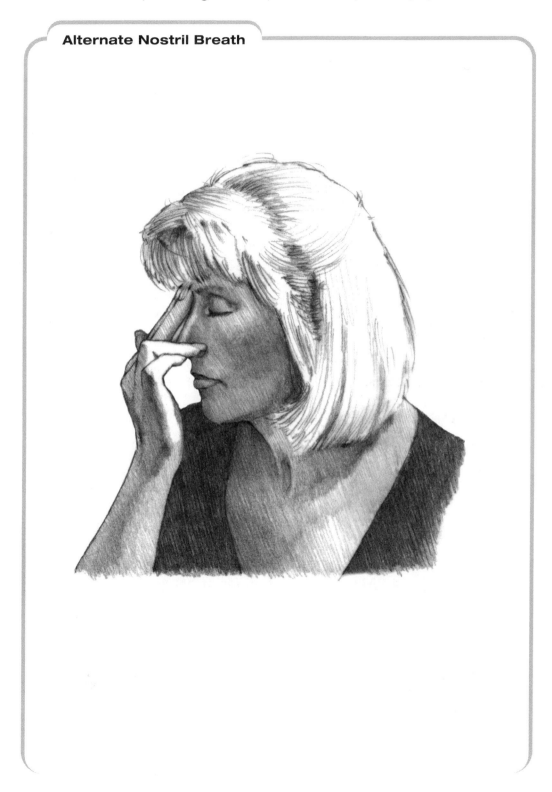

WEIGHT GAIN

Weight gain during menopause is not a necessary outcome of aging, because with a regular exercise program and limiting food intake, you can maintain your weight as you age. The hormones that change during menopause may include the ones responsible for appetite, so many women find that they want to eat more than usual. This is fine, as long as your exercise level also increases at the same time. Because this time of life is often a time of emotional upheaval for many women who experience major lifestyle changes, it can often be easy to indulge in "comfort eating." Concerns about body image and aging are uppermost in the minds of many 40-plus women at this age, and yoga has much to offer. Rather than encourage yo-yo dieting, or the latest choreographed fad in exercise programs, yoga uses ancient, scientifically proven methods of working from the inside out to correct imbalances that are causing the weight gain.

These yogic techniques work to speed up the metabolic rate by increasing oxygen levels needed to combust food. They tone the muscles in the abdomen that move food through the gut, so that the elimination system works effectively and constipation does not occur. Constipation causes fluid retention and consequent weight gain. Most importantly, the visualization exercises create and refine a perfect self-image for the mind to work from, rather than reinforcing an old, negative image. Without a clear mental image of the way a person wants to eventually look after weight loss, the mind will not have a clear blueprint for producing the desired outcome.

Visualize: In any self-improvement program, whether giving up smoking, exercising more, or losing weight, it is important to see yourself as you would really like to be, and not to dwell on the way you are now, with all your limitations and faults. It is also important to keep reinforcing this positive self-image, by regularly refining it, to reflect on the way you want to be, until it is perfect. Take time to think about how you would like to look, speak, and interact with others. If at first, you cannot see a clear image, then reflect on these things, and eventually you will be able to visualize your perfect self-image. Know that if you give your mind a blueprint, which says, "I am too fat," or lazy, or stupid, or whatever, then your mind will produce a body to go with that blueprint. But if you give your mind a perfect blueprint of exactly the way you want to become, it will have a very clear image from which it can work. Realize that you must first see in order to become. Visualize yourself aging well, with your weight under control, so that you can eventually forget about it, and begin to work on the higher aspects of yourself. See yourself with a healthy, strong, and flexible body, a focused mind, and an open heart.

11. Metabolic Workout

This series of four simple exercises takes a mere 10 minutes to complete. It is based on an ancient yogic series of postures that promote youth and vitality. It works to balance the metabolic rate and energy levels of each of the major endocrine glands in the body, which control many functions. The chakras corresponding to these glands are often depicted visually as vortices of whirling energy. The yogis say that if the energy in each of these chakra centers rotates at the same speed and direction, perfect health will be restored. It is only when these energy centers become sluggish or overactive that ill health occurs.

Exercise 1

Benefits: This exercise activates the thyroid gland in the throat, which controls energy levels and activates the reproductive glands in the groin.

Focus: on keeping your hips on the ground, and on squeezing your chin firmly onto your throat.

Note: If this exercise causes you any lower back pain, try bending your legs first, before extending them to the ceiling, or making a fist under each buttock before lifting your legs.

1. Lie on your back, with your palms flat on the floor, beside your thighs.

2. Inhale, and bring your legs straight up to right angles with the floor.

3. At the same time, lift your head and squeeze your chin onto your chest.

4. Exhale through your mouth, and lower your head and legs to the floor.

5. Repeat seven times.

Exercise 2

Benefit: This posture activates the adrenals in the lower back, which control stress levels, and the thyroid in the throat which controls energy levels, as the chin is squeezed onto the chest. The adrenals also produce estrogen-like substances at menopause to offset naturally falling levels in the body.

Focus: on pinching your shoulder blades together, and dropping your head right back, to create a strong lock over the thyroid in your throat. Also focus on arching backward strongly, to squeeze the adrenals on top of your kidneys.

1. Kneel on the floor, with your buttocks off your heels and your toes tucked under.

Metabolic Workout—Exercises 1 and 2

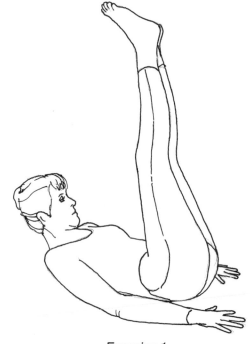

Exercise 1

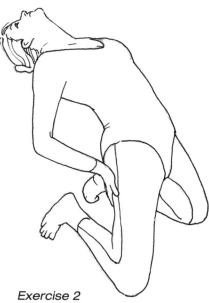

Exercise 2

2. Place your palms flat against the back of your thighs.

3. Inhale through your nose, and lean backward.

4. Arch your back, push your hips forward, and drop your head back, stretching through the throat center.

5. Exhale through your mouth, and return to the start, bringing your chin firmly onto your chest.

6. Repeat seven times.

7. Release, by sitting between your heels, with your head to the floor.

Exercise 3

Benefits: This exercise tightens and tones up the abdominal muscles, which can make the stomach appear flatter. It tones the pelvic floor area and prevents incontinence as we age. It also prevents wetting ourselves when we sneeze or do star jumps at the gym. It strengthens the muscles and bones in the arms and upper body, as well as the legs. In addition, it activates the parathyroids in the neck, which control calcium levels in the blood.

Focus: on pinching your buttock and stomach muscles tightly together, to strengthen your pelvic floor area. Use the strength of your thighs to keep pushing your hips higher into the air and improve the position.

1. Sit on the floor, with your legs apart, palms beside your hips and your fingertips facing outward. Rest your chin on your chest.

2. Inhale through your nose, bend your knees, lift your hips, and squeeze your buttock muscles tightly.

3. Pinch your shoulder blades together, and drop your head right back.

4. Push into the pads of your hands and feet, to keep your hips high and your back arched.

5. Exhale through your mouth, and return your hips to the floor. Straighten your legs, and put your chin back onto your chest.

6. Repeat seven times.

7. Release, by lying on the floor and breathing deeply.

Exercise 4

Benefits: This posture activates the thyroid gland in the throat, for high energy levels, as your head is arched back and then squeezed onto your chest. It also allows extra blood flow to your brain, without having to push against gravity. It puts pressure on the pituitary in the brain, which controls many body functions, including appetite. It also controls the pineal, which regulates moods, and moods can play a major part in the success of any weight-reduction program. It strengthens the muscles and bones of the forearms and upper body, as it bears the total body weight in the inverted position.

Focus: on keeping your hands and feet in the same position throughout the exercise, and on pushing your buttocks high into the air with each inverted "V" position. Keep your head well through your shoulders, and push up from the pads of your hands, to move your weight back into your heels.

1. Lie on your stomach, with your legs wide and your toes tucked under.

2. Bend your elbows, and place your forearms beside your upper chest, with fingers outstretched.

3. Arch your upper body off the floor, and straighten your arms, supporting your upper body on your outstretched arms. Your pelvis should still be on the floor.

4. Inhale, and pushing onto your hands and toes, and lift your hips into an inverted "V" shape.

5. Push your head through your shoulders, and squeeze your chin onto your chest. Stretch, and lengthen through your spine.

6. Exhale through your mouth, and move your weight back into your hands. Arching your spine, drop your pelvis back to the starting position on the floor.

8. Straighten your elbows, and arch your spine and head back.

9. Repeat seven times.

This series of simple exercises is excellent for activating the metabolic rate, first thing in the morning, and for providing an even flow of energy throughout the day.

Begin with seven repetitions of each of the four exercises. Add one repetition each day to each of the exercises, until you can do each exercise rapidly 21 times. This will take around 15 to 20 minutes to complete, and can be done as slowly or quickly as desired. Maximum benefit for weight loss will be obtained by completing each exercise 21 times. Do not be surprised if people begin to comment on how well you look, and say you look younger. Energetic

Metabolic Workout—Exercises 3 and 4

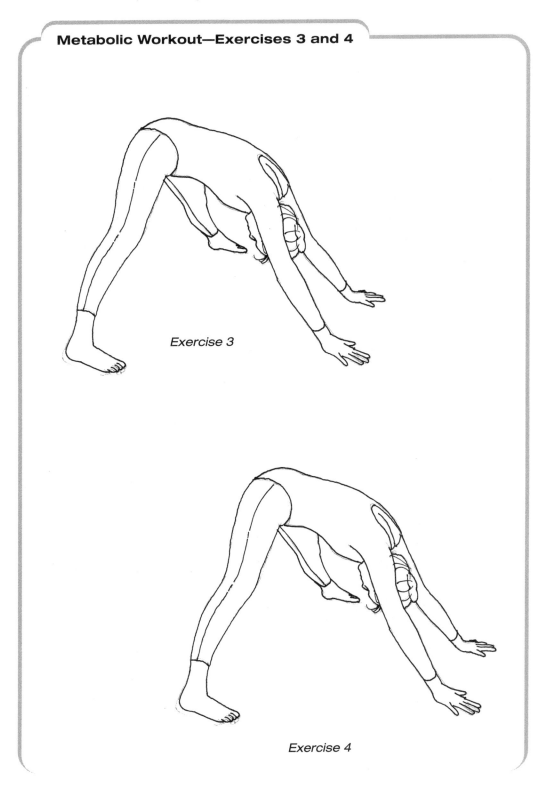

Exercise 3

Exercise 4

people always appear to be younger than those who are more sluggish. The combination of a clear image of the desired outcome, plus increased energy levels, will result in weight reduction over time.

12. Shoulder Stand with Heels Together

Benefits: This posture improves the levels of oxygen in the blood stream to speed up the metabolic rate for the combustion of food. It balances the thyroid gland, so the metabolic rate is neither too speedy, nor too sluggish for improved digestion and metabolism of food. It improves the blood circulation to the brain for clear thinking, and promotes clear healthy skin and shiny hair.

Focus: on keeping your weight evenly balanced over both shoulder blades, and on breathing deeply through your diaphragm and upper chest area, to steady the posture. Feel a lightness in your body, and visualize that, in time, any excess weight will metabolize and leave you feeling both lighter and younger.

1. Lie on your back, with your feet up the wall and your buttocks touching the wall.

2. Bend your knees, and place your feet hip-width apart on the wall. Your hands should be beside your hips, with your palms flat.

3. Inhale, and push your feet against the wall, while arching your back, moving your body weight into the top of your shoulder blades.

4. Support your waist with your hands, and with your fingertips turned in toward your spine.

5. Move your weight from side to side, to bring your body weight as high as possible onto your shoulders.

6. Move your elbows close together behind your back for support, and breathe slowly, to steady your body.

7. Keeping your spine strong and arched, lift one foot of the wall and straighten your leg.

8. Take your weight onto the top of your shoulders, slowly lift your other leg off the wall, and straighten. Do not move your head or neck in this position.

9. Rest your chin on your chest, to create a lock over your throat and restrict the circulation to your thyroid gland.

10. Bring the soles of your feet together, bend your knees, and bring your feet into the groin.

Shoulder Stand with Heels Together

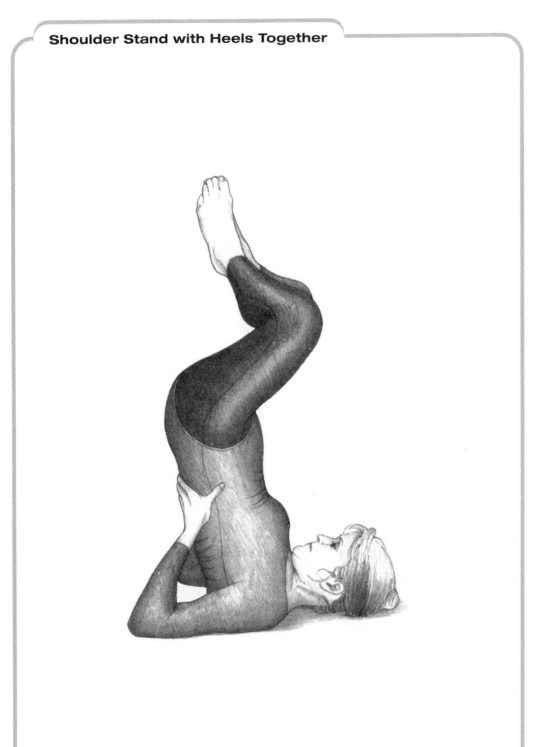

11. Straighten up through your back, and breathe slowly seven times.

12. To release, extend your legs to the ceiling. Bend one knee and place your foot back on the wall. Then return your other foot to the wall.

13. Slide your elbows out, and lower your hips to the floor. Rest your legs up the wall. The thyroid gland is now flushed with fresh, oxygenated blood, as the lock over your throat is released.

13. Extended Banda

This Bandha holds the stomach lock for longer periods of time, to strengthen the intestinal muscles. Food can then be moved quickly through the elimination system. If these muscles become slack, food is kept in the gut for longer periods of time, where it putrefies, because of the moist, warm environment. Water is retained, to dilute the toxins. This causes fluid retention, bloating and weight gain.

Benefits: This exercise greatly improves the tone and strength of the muscles of the abdomen to move digested food out of the elimination system efficiently. Constipation always makes the body feel heavy. This posture relieves constipation, by improving the functioning of the elimination system to prevent bloating.

Focus: on keeping your chin tucked into your throat and your stomach pulled in tightly, creating a strong vacuum over the pancreas, to massage all of your internal organs, particularly the pancreas which controls sugar levels in the body.

1. Stand with your legs wide apart.

2. Bend your knees and squat, with your hands resting on your knees and your fingertips facing inward.

3. Inhale, and exhale forcefully through your open mouth.

4. Close your mouth, tuck your chin into your chest, and hold the breath.

5. Suck the stomach muscles back up and under the rib cage and hold your breath for the count of seven.

6. To release, exhale, and straighten your legs. Bend forward, and hang loosely.

7. Repeat, but hold your breath for 14 counts, and then release.

8. Repeat a third time, holding your breath for 21 counts, before releasing, by hanging loosely like a rag doll.

Extended Banda

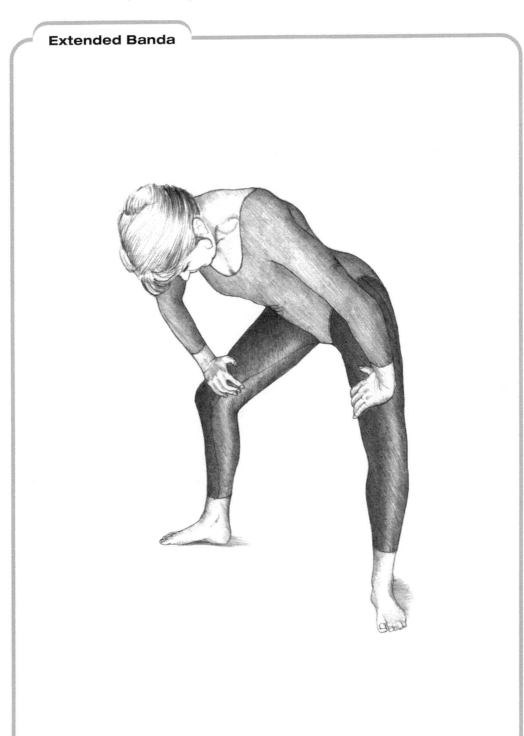

THE IMPORTANCE OF DRINKING WATER FOR WEIGHT LOSS

Drinking plenty of fresh plain water is recommended in any weight loss plan, but other than for clear skin and a lack of cellulite, has anyone ever explained why? The more important reason involves maintaining a healthy elimination system, which is a key feature of our health and well-being, and an essential element in weight-loss programs.

Question: *Why do we need to replace fluids lost from the body by drinking plenty of water?*

Answer: Our bodies are mostly made up of fluids. These fluids need to be replaced daily because:

♦ Approximately three pints of water per day are lost through the kidneys.

♦ Approximately one pint of water per day is lost through the skin in perspiration.

♦ A further pint is lost through breathing and vaporization.

Question: *What happens if we do not replace this lost fluid in our bodies on a daily basis?*

Answer: The body will seek out the replacement fluids it needs from the undigested sludge sitting in the intestines, waiting to be eliminated.

Question: *What effect will that have on the body?*

Answer: As water is withdrawn from this sludge, the fecal matter becomes harder, resulting in constipation. The body will retain water to dilute these toxic substances and bloating and weight gain will occur. Because the water from the undigested sludge is dirty, when it is recirculated throughout the body, it will increase the toxins in the body. This can lead to feelings of tiredness and lethargy, and the body will be more vulnerable to infection.

Question: *How many glasses of water should we drink every day? How can we increase our daily intake?*

Answer:

♦ Drink two glasses of water first thing in the morning and last thing at night, as a reminder.

♦ Carry water in your car, and keep a glass at your desk, so you can sip throughout the day. The amount of water you consume will soon add up to the recommended 8 to10 glasses a day.

♦ Replace soft drinks and cordials with plain, room-temperature water.

♦ Aim to increase your daily intake slowly, over time, and be prepared to urinate more frequently, as your body flushes out toxins.

Question: *What are the benefits?*

Answer: You will experience greater feelings of well-being, fewer illnesses, an increase in your energy level, fewer weight problems, and a healthy digestive system that is free of constipation.

Full Yoga Breath

The Full Yoga Breath is also an excellent way to increase the oxygen levels in the blood, increasing the metabolic rate to help combust food. Follow the instructions given in Chapter 2: Getting Started. Practice the Full Yoga Breath regularly in bed, at morning and night, so that it will become easier to practice in an upright position throughout the day.

DISRUPTED SLEEP PATTERNS

Menopause is often a time of major family upheaval, with children leaving home and elderly parents needing more attention. It is not unusual for sleep patterns to be disturbed at this stage of life.

The parathyroids in the side of the neck play a major role in getting a good night's sleep, because they regulate calcium levels in the body, for strong healthy nerves and bones. When these glands are healthy and function as they should, they ensure that sufficient calcium reaches the bloodstream for calm nerves. The Seated Fish posture illustrated below creates a lock over these glands and helps to maintain calcium balance. As the head is inverted, pressure is put on the pituitary gland, which acts like a feedback system for many other glands in the body, including the ones that regulate our sleep patterns.

14. The Seated Fish

Benefits: The Seated Fish not only works on balancing calcium levels for healthy nerves and a good night's sleep, but on strengthening the bones of the wrist and arms. It also puts pressure on the pituitary, which regulates sleep patterns.

Focus: on pushing on your hands, to improve the arch in your back, and on letting your head just hang, to improve the lock over your parathyroids.

1. Sit with your legs outstretched, and your palms beside your hips on the floor.

2. Inhale, then exhale, and lift your hips off the floor.

3. Arch your back strongly, and let your head hang between your shoulders.

4. Push your toes flat to the floor to support your body.

Seated Fish

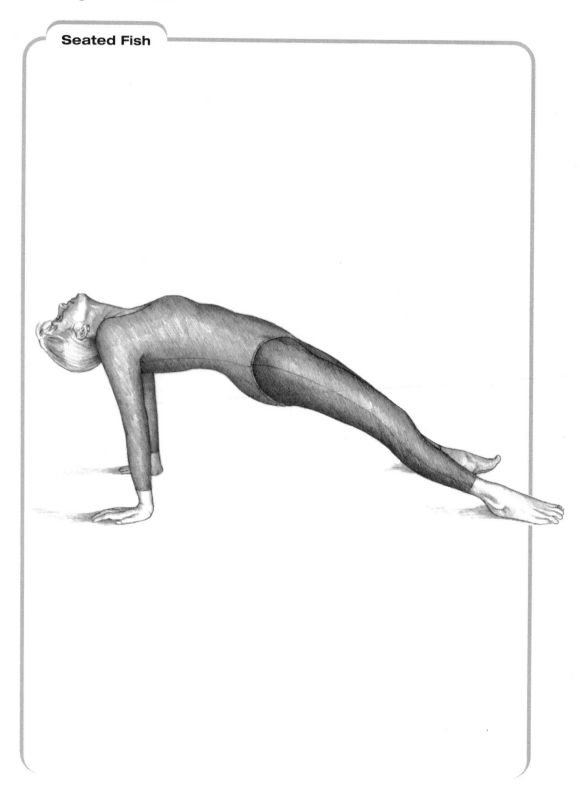

5. Keep your elbows locked, and push on your hands, to support your entire body weight.

6. Breathe slowly seven times.

7. To return, lower your hips to the floor, lie down, and rest with your feet flopped apart and your palms facing upward.

Rhythmic Breathing

One of the simplest ways to top up your "sleep bank" is to take an afternoon cat nap, using deep, rhythmic yoga breathing to induce a short, relaxing sleep. Lie on a bed in a darkened room, and begin seven rounds of Full Yoga Breath (FYB). (See Chapter 2: Getting Started for instructions for FYB). Release the technique, but if necessary, complete another seven rounds. More than likely, this will be sufficient to allow you to drift off into a relaxing state for a short catnap.

At night, deep, rhythmic breathing is one of the simplest ways to induce a good night's sleep, as the mind finds this is very soothing and comforting. When we are tired and irritable, we tend to breathe erratically, which irritates the mind and disturbs sleep. When we can't get to sleep, we feel anxious, and our breathing patterns become more erratic, leading to less chance of falling asleep. Practicing deep, rhythmic breathing before sleeping—and during the night if you wake up—is a simple way to break the cycle of sleeplessness. And it's much better than a sleeping pill! If you suffer from insomnia on a regular basis, be patient with these techniques, as it will take time to undo poor sleeping habits. The Sukra Breath described here is an easy breath to practice at night, because you can do it lying down. Begin with seven rounds of Sukra Breath, then release the technique, and lie quietly. Repeating the Sukra Breath for another seven rounds will normally induce sound sleep.

15. Sukra Breath

The Sukra Breath, or "sweet breath" induces a calming rhythm in the mind, which is conducive to sleep.

Benefits: It improves the depth and rhythm of the breath, stills all those busy thoughts in the mind, and calms the emotions, to induce a good night's sleep.

Focus: on making your inhalations the same length as your exhalations.

Visualize: See yourself making peace with the past, peace with the future, and being at peace with the present. As you drop off to sleep, say to yourself, "I am giving in and letting go of all those things in my life that are now finished, that have had their time, and that may be taking up my best energies." In this way, you can make space in your mind for new opportunities, relationships, and ideas to come into your life. Before dropping off to sleep, repeat to yourself, "I am giving in more . . . and more . . . and more deeply . . ."

1. Lie on your back, with your hands loosely by your side and your palms upward.

2. Allow your feet to flop apart.

3. Lift your eyebrows, and smooth out your forehead, releasing any tension in your face. Unlock your jaw, releasing any tension, and let your mouth be soft.

4. Imagine that you have a white square in your mind, made of fluorescent tubing.

5. Move your attention to the bottom left-hand corner of the square. Inhale slowly for the count of four, and imagine moving up the left side of the square.

7. Keep your attention on the top of the left corner of the square.

8. Hold your breath for the count of four, as you imagine moving across to the top, right-hand side of the square.

9. Exhale for the count of four, as you imagine moving down from the top right corner to the bottom right corner of the square.

10. Hold your breath for four counts, as you return to the left side of the square.

11. This completes one round. Repeat seven rounds, keeping your concentration on moving around the square.

16. Candle Meditation

The art of staying in the present and focusing all our energies and thoughts on the now is a skill that is well worth learning. Meditating on a regular basis is the key to this process. Use this meditation before going to bed, to focus on the light within, to bring you back into the moment, and to still your mind before sleeping.

Albert Schweitzer once said, "The only essential thing is that we strive to have light in ourselves. Others will recognize our striving, and when people have light in themselves, it radiates out to others. Then we get to know each other, as we walk together in the darkness, without needing to pass our hands over each other's faces or to intrude into each others hearts."

Very often this light within us is swamped by personal darkness all around us, in the form of a lack of vision and direction for our lives, crushed values, lack of familial patterns, dead ethics, and no personal responsibility. But light reveals the loveliest things hidden in the darkness—for example, a diamond, an opal or a crystal. As you practice this meditation, imagine it revealing all those wonderful aspects of yourself, such as your sense of loyalty, love, devotion and honesty.

Benefits: Sitting still doing nothing for 20 to 30 minutes, once or twice a day, automatically harmonizes all the body's vital biorhythms. It also gives the mind a better rest that even sleep cannot provide. During sleep, the mind often wanders in a chaotic dreamland that leaves it more exhausted than before sleep. By contrast, meditation stills the mind, drains it of mental clutter, and leaves it thoroughly revitalized.

Focus: on just letting your thoughts come and go in a very detached way, rather than trying to stop them. Let the light of the flame symbolize the light within you that will dispel the outer darkness. Feel yourself beginning to radiate the light—a light that gives you courage, strength—and the will to keep going when the going gets tough.

To begin:

Light a candle (scented or unscented) in your favorite darkened room. If possible, sit comfortably on the floor, in a cross-legged position. Alternatively, sit on the floor with your legs outstretched, and lean against a firm surface, or sit in a chair with the candle at table height. Place the candle a few feet away from your body.

1. Allow your eyes to rest on the flame without staring. Look deeply into the flame, taking note of its color, shape, sound and smell.

2. Imagine being filled with this light, deep in every cell of your body, and radiating it to others around you.

3. Begin seven rounds of Sukra Breathing.

4. Allow your logical thoughts to subside and the chatter in your mind to be still.

5. Watch your thoughts coming and going in a very detached way.

6. Be aware of your breath coming and going effortlessly.

7. Be aware of your posture settling into a relaxed state.

8. Allow yourself to settle into the stillness descending over you.

9. Now, close your eyes gently, and imagine drawing the image of the light deep within your heart, so that it illuminates all the

wonderful qualities within you that often get overlooked in the business of the day, including your sense of compassion and forgiveness, loyalty, devotion, strength, and courage.

10. Stay focused on that inner vision of light within you, as you silently repeat to yourself three times:

> *I am in the light*
>
> *I am of the light*
>
> *I am the Light*

Now, simply allow yourself to listen in the stillness of your own being for approximately 10 to 15 minutes. When you are ready to return, deepen your breath slowly, and begin to stretch your body. With minimum movement and effort, prepare for bed and look forward to a deep, relaxing sleep.

Note: The art of meditation is both universal and personal. No single recipe promises to be perfect for everyone, so do not be discouraged if you do not experience the inner stillness initially. You cannot stop all those annoying thoughts coming into your mind, but you can choose not to be distracted by them, and move back down into the silence. With practice, you will learn to be aware when your mind wanders, to be less and less distracted, and to be more detached in watching these thoughts.

Sometimes it helps to use a candle, soft music, or aromatherapy oils to create the conditions for meditative stillness to occur, so that we can enter that dream-like state where we experience the art of simply being. This exercise, using a candle to maintain focus and concentration, is but a tool for learning the deeper levels of meditation, which will come with practice. Eventually, these props will not be necessary, and you will be able to drift into a meditative state naturally and easily, just by using rhythmic breathing to focus your mind.

Remember that the secret of meditation is patience . . . and still more patience.

Conclusion

After reading this book, you will realize that osteoporosis does not have to be an expected outcome of aging, and that if you expect to remain strong in old age and put your energy behind that thought, then you will.

The strong correlation between hatha yoga and the prevention of osteoporosis cannot be ignored. Yoga creates a balanced harmony between the ovaries, adrenals, parathyroids, pituitary and pineal gland, ensuring that the body receives a steady supply of the right hormones for maintaining bone strength and maximum health and well-being. The regular practice of weight-bearing hatha yoga postures offers women everywhere a safe, scientifically proven way to build bone strength and avoid this debilitating disease.

There is perhaps no better example of how important strong weight-bearing exercise is for preventing osteoporosis than the case of film star, Christopher Reeve. On May 27, 1995, he fell from a horse, becoming instantly quadriplegic. He faced a future of muscular atrophy, loss of bone density, and the early onset of osteoporosis. Yet because Reeve believes so strongly that he will one day walk again, he has put himself through a relentless, daily physical exercise program since the accident. He knows that, in the event of a possible cure, he can only be a candidate if the muscles in his legs and arms do not atrophy.

During the summer of 1998, he was tested for a new "walking therapy." Placed in a parachute harness, his body was lifted by an overhead hoist onto an ordinary treadmill. When the treadmill moved, Reeve exercised his leg muscles and put ligaments, tendons, and bones into motion, while experiencing a good cardiovascular workout. The theory behind this is that the spinal cord has a memory and apparently, despite damage, enough connections remain to generate the mechanics of walking.

As Reeve was hoisted into position and the treadmill set in motion, his right leg moved back, his hip transferred the weight to his left leg, and moved forward in a regular walking motion. This meant that all of the exercising he had done had really paid off. What's more, three and a half years after his accident, his bone density tested 20% higher than ten other individuals of the same weight, height, age, and general physical condition. Reeve attributes this outcome partially to genetics, but more importantly, to the benefits of diet and daily physical exercise.

Let this example be like a guiding light within you, and know that you, too, can use the power of your mind and the strength of your body to age as well as possible, for as long as possible.